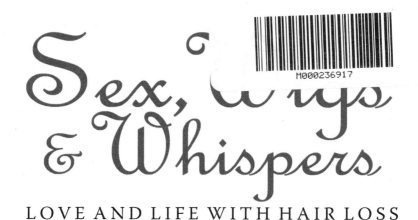

Sex, Wigs & Whispers

LOVE AND LIFE WITH HAIR LOSS

M000236917

AMY GIBSON

Sex, Wigs and Whispers
Copyright © 2015 by Amy Gibson

Published by CreatedHair Media
Los Angeles, California
www.createdhair.com
877-926-9300

All Rights Reserved. Excerpt as permitted under the United States Copyright Act of 1976, no part of this publication may be reproduced or distributed in any form, or by any means, or stored in a database retrieval system, without the prior written permission of the copyright holder, except by a reviewer, who may quote brief passages in review. The scanning, uploading, and distribution of this book via the Internet or via any other means without the permission of the publisher is illegal and punishable by law. Purchase only authorized electronic editions, and do not participate in or encourage electronic piracy of copyrighted materials.

Neither the publisher nor the author is engaged in rendering professional advice or services to the individual reader. The ideas, procedures, and suggestions contained in this book are not intended as a substitute for consulting with a medical professional or counselor. All matters regarding your health and wellness. Neither the author nor the publisher shall be liable or responsible for any loss, injury, or damage allegedly arising from any information or suggestion in this book. The opinions expressed in this book represent the personal views of the author, and are for informational purposes only. This book is not intended to replace counseling advice, diagnosis, treatment, or other therapeutic intervention by a qualified professional.

ISBN 978-0-9862842-3-6 - Hard Cover
ISBN 978-0-9862842-4-3 - Perfectbound
ISBN 978-0-9862842-5-0 - ePub

Edited by: Bill Quateman
Cover Photography: Raul Vega
Illustrations by: Juan Carlos Diaz
Cover Design: Bill Fate
Interior Design and Layout: Kimberly Leonard
Hair: Celebrity Stylist Kathleen Leonard
Makeup: Tamara Ogden

Dedication

To all women and children who are living with hair loss
and fighting to find a way to hold on to their essence.

To all women fighting for their own voice and presence
in a world that so easily tries to silence it.

Acknowledgments

To God. Thank you for always bringing me what is needed at the perfect time to do the work you have asked me to do here in this lifetime. It's not always easy, but this work has brought me more joy, more love, more humility and deeper insight, that I could have ever imagined.

To Bill; your unstoppable support and absolute unconditional love and acceptance of who I am as a woman, a bald sexy woman, is what has propelled me to finish this book. Thank you for your incredible help, your editing talents, your deep insight and hours of hard work. I love you and am so grateful to be in this life with you.

To my extraordinary mother Tobe; who gave me the strength and insight over the years to understand my own "I AM", even when I was certain it never existed. Thank you for teaching me to never let anything or anyone stop me from my dreams. I miss you, Mom. I also know you're with me, on every page I have written.

To my dad, Robert; I will always love you, even though many may not understand how I can. Thank you for all things you instilled in me that helped me become the strong woman I am.

To my sister, Jody; who has taught me the art of patience and true forgiveness. Thank you for your immense help with finishing this important book. Thank you for accepting my artistry without judgment and allowing me to be who I have needed to be here.

To Dylan and India; thank you for putting up with all my papers!

To Hope Mineo; you are truly one of the most gifted, phenomenal women I have met on this plane. Your level of integrity shines though, as does your light. Thank you for your beautiful help in bringing this dream to life.

To Kathleen; my associate, wonderful stylist, and dear friend; Thank you for taking this ride with me for so many years to help those in need.

To Juan; thank you for your immense love, support, and for sharing your beautiful spirit. Thank you for loaning me your brilliant hands to bring these women to life with such precision.

To Bill Fate; Thank you for your generous help and beautiful talent over the years.

To John Arno; Thank you for always being there for me. Your tremendous generosity, love and support, in all areas of my life touch my core in ways that transcend our 'agreement.'

To Kim Leonard; Thank you for going beyond the call of duty. The immense caring and patience you have shown me and my "baby" has put me in tears many a time after our calls.

To some of my greatest listeners.... LillyPoo, Punum, Mr. Big, Hanna, and My Harry. You fill my heart.

To Nita, Lori, Farryl, Twink, Rona, Gail, Murray, Parrot Face, Georgia, My Mochi, Amy B., Megs, and all my friends and wonderful clients, who for so many years, have supported my desires and dreams to bring this book to women all over the world. I thank you for your everlasting patient ears and unselfish hearts.

Table of Contents

Preface

Since the beginning of time hair has been a source of strength, magic and beauty, in both fantasy and reality...

Adolescence can exuberant and a wonderful time of curiosity; at the same time it can be awkward, marked with insecurities, a longing to fit in and a loathing of almost everything that exists. Adolescents' physical bodies and emotions change like rapid fire, waging war with themselves and often everyone around them. In the best of circumstances adolescence is a time of discomfort, distress, anxiety and longing.

This is when I lost my hair!

The things in my life that would have normally 'calmed' me in this tumultuous journey of growing up – sports, family, acting, friends and my long flowing hair, were marred by fear of someone discovering my bald patches, lies to cast mates and friends, a highly dysfunctional family and the devastation of my perception that I was no longer whole or beautiful.

In the beginning, and as years went on, I stayed away from sports, the beach and hanging with friends… because something as simple as the wind could give me away.

As a soap opera star, I kept my distance from co-workers and the press for fear of being ousted from the industry as a bald freak. At that time, baldness was a shameful subject that was never discussed. Dating was impossible, because books with insights like this did not exist; nor was it possible to get help about how to be normal in a world that worships hair.

Eventually, lack of self-esteem consumed and ruled me. I left the entertainment industry.

Holding onto the tiny bit of self-confidence I had left presented a tremendous challenge when I became a business executive, with nowhere to turn for help or support about how to fit in, as I still struggled with having no hair in a world of people with flowing locks.

Today, as a successful wig and accessories designer, speaker and personal hair loss consultant for over 15 years, I have learned there is a different and better way to grow up with and live, with hair loss. And I have worked continuously to help women and children from all over the world face their hair loss journey with power and grace.

Now I am grateful for the opportunity to show others what has worked for me and how I've found peace of mind; using practical solutions, a smile, a sense of humor, spiritual guidance and an attitude that inspires from within. This creates a true transformation. I have successfully used these and many tools I'll be showing you during intimacy and in all areas of my life, and they have worked. They can, and will – work for you too.

If you're reading this book, you likely wear alternative hair (wigs, extensions, top pieces, etc.) or know someone who does. Maybe you were drawn to the title and are simply curious. If you're facing hair loss, maybe you're looking for answers and a way to live a full life in the midst of dealing with your lack of or disappearing hair. Maybe you've been searching for a way to feel comfortable with sex and dating with your wig, but have not had the tools or confidence to do so. For many of you, maybe you want guidance, support and to learn how to get in touch with your sensuality again after your hair loss.

Whatever brought you here – welcome to my world; where you will now be in control of your choices, your emotions, your look, your inner beauty and most of all... your power.

What I will share with you first hand is that I have been on this hair loss journey for thirty years; I have walked in your shoes. I have felt the pain, the fear, the disappointments, the hurts, the tears, the devastation, the embarrassments, shame, confusion, guilt and the crushing loneliness – just like you have.

Absolutely and without a shadow of a doubt, it is possible, doable and expected, that after you read this book you will have the tools to live – even with your hair loss – a full and empowered life. You'll be able to enjoy intimacy on all levels – wherever and whenever you want it… on your own terms.

I am extremely raw, candid, direct and transparent in this 'Book of Revelations.' I do so not to offend; but to share my journey and open up possibilities that you dare dream possible. You have a front row seat to intimate details of my life and I let you in as close as possible without you actually being there. Much of what is on these pages I have never discussed with anyone, including best friends, lovers or family. However, I felt that if I were going to truly help and make a difference for the people I know that are out there facing this – I needed to come clean.

This book is full of the lies I told to help me keep my hair loss secret throughout twenty years in television, a painful and devastating family secret, rape and many more incidents from my life, shared – so if any of you have had any similar experiences, these pages are intended to help you move forward in your life and find your own personal peace. Much of this book has been painful to write; forcing me to take a look at my own challenges that to my surprise were still present.

You will get answers and strategies, so that you have an entirely new perspective on the woman you have been, the woman you are now, and the woman you wish to become.

xiv

This will allow you to make powerful choices for yourself; free from the fears you have been living with and that have possibly been running your life. Now, you can learn about the techniques I created over the years to help me successfully handle any intimate situation. With these useful tips, you will once again be able to enjoy a beautiful romance without any emotional distractions or attachments, and without anyone discovering your secret – unless you want them to know.

There are many scenarios that I have experienced with men, good and bad, covered in this book that I have overcome. Some are humorous. Others tug at the heart. Either way, you will remember your own experiences and gain new skills about how to be behave differently in the same situations.

Sex, Wigs, and Whispers will show you how to discover (or reconnect with) your own power, use that power, and how to hold onto it in the midst of extreme vulnerability.

Wearing 'created hair' can be both wonderful and frightening. Wonderful, because you can be anyone you want to be; frightening, because of its unknown territory.

However, by the time we're through this won't be such a huge concern for you anymore, because you will know what to do, how to say it and who to say it to. That is, of course, if you choose to.

My intention with this book has more to do with being comfortable in your own power regardless of whether you have hair or not. If you are fine without wearing hair and feel beautiful, sensual and solid in your core, then I support your decision. Bless you, you're beautiful.

You'll soon understand that I am all about choice and nothing is more powerful than giving yourself the ability to choose. Once a woman chooses to find her essence again she can handle her hair loss much easier. When she re-establishes her ability to accept her own sexuality and sensuality once again, she can truly be anyone she chooses to be. Then the world is her oyster. May you find your pearl in my book.

NOTE: **The Pearl Program is what this book is based on. Women have flown in from all over the world to spend a day learning these techniques.**

Introduction

INTENTION AND THE POWER OF CHOICE

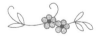

For every beauty there is an eye somewhere to see it. For every truth there is an ear somewhere to hear it. For every love there is a heart somewhere to receive it.

Ivan Panin

I learned early on about life's challenges, setting my intentions and the power of choice.

My overall intention has been to live life full out, regardless of its challenges and to do all I can to help others do the same. My focus has been women with hair loss from any disease or treatment, including Alopecia and chemotherapy.

Sadly, below is how the hair loss journey begins for most women.

Thoughts and fears about your hair loss leave you plagued before you even drift off to sleep. You never miss a mirror; like a spy on a mission, making certain your hair is covering that bald spot or thinning area. There are those of you who will never even look in the mirror because you can't handle what you see. And this is just when you're alone. Being with other people, especially the opposite sex brings with it a whole new set of fears.

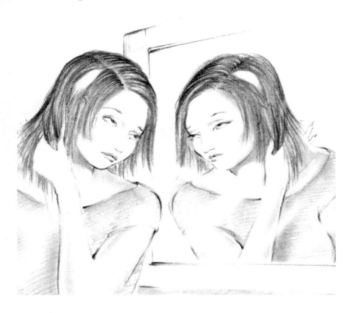

My intention is that as you read this book you say to yourself:

'Is this me? Do I really do this? Is that what he was thinking when I did that? Wow! I'm going to use that one!'

Sex, Wigs and Whispers

Let's face it, the subject of hair loss, or being intimate and having sex with a wig on, are not exactly something we've been introduced to in school or something our dear ole' mom sat us down to discuss! Until recently, most of us have associated wigs with illness. Thanks to celebrities like Lady Gaga, Madonna, Cher, and Jessica Simpson, 'alternative hair' has become more common in the past few years. But if any of these women have a wig mishap, they are not running for cover hiding bald spots or worse, a barren head.

Many other questions may likely pop up for you:

How do we wear a wig correctly so we can keep our secret?

How do we live our lives like other normal women who are interacting in social events, participating in sports, dancing, and dating with this foreign object on our heads – without anyone knowing?

Regardless of how gorgeous your piece may be, if it looks like a wig and you act like it's a wig, guess what – everyone will know it's a wig!

Have you ever been on a date and its going great; then that 'time' finally arrives for the romantic kiss. He reaches his hand behind your neck and you suddenly get that awful feeling in the pit of your stomach. Your heart starts pounding, your adrenalin rises, your hands begin to sweat, and you hear nothing your date says because your mind is going 100 MPH thinking,

"Oh My God he knows!"

You're sure he's going to freak, ask lots of questions, and then he's going to run and never want to see you again?!

Sound familiar?

This book gives you the tools you need to handle this anxiety if it arises and helps you avoid that fearful place again.

Have you ever been in bed with your lover and in the midst of the hottest moment, gone into a panic because you don't know how to stop him from touching or 'pulling' your hair without bringing attention to your secret?

I have.

The ideas in this book put you in the driver's seat; they will show you the ways to keep these circumstances from throwing you, using subtle movements that he'll never catch onto and alleviate the anxiety so you can remain relaxed and in control... and have fun.

Have you ever refused a simple walk on the beach on a beautiful day with your date – simply out of fear that the wind will expose your wig?

However, there are distinct ways to use your body that will help you avoid such circumstances from happening which are covered in this book.

How about not wearing the perfect hat because of the heavy perspiration it creates with your wig? I'm right there with you!

Have you ever gone out on a date and suddenly been faced with a spontaneous convertible ride, instead of that coupe you were expecting? Then freaked out that your wig was going to fly off? One of my more interesting moments...

No worries, this book introduces you to wonderful products that you can use at a moment's notice to help keep you in your power!

Have you ever made excuses for not taking a Jacuzzi, or showering with your lover – all because you were scared to get your wig wet?

Sex, Wigs and Whispers

Ever pass on swimming with your boyfriend or a group of friends, even in 90-degree weather because you were afraid your hair would come off in the water?

This was a tough one...

No problem. With the easy-to-follow processes laid out in this book, you'll be playfully and sensually gliding through the water again. You see, all of the above (and many more), is what it was like for me for years; until I figured out the simple ways in which to navigate many of these challenges.

Have you wondered?

Do I tell him? Is he ready? What if he can't handle it? Will he leave me?

This book will help you learn to understand your own actions and how to trust your instincts on a deeper level. You will come to know what is really propelling you to tell him and most importantly, if it's coming from an organic place or out of need; something you will learn to see quickly and avoid. You'll know exactly:

1) Is he *worthy* of your **secret?**

2) Is he *ready* to **hear** your **secret?**

3) Are you *ready* to **tell him** your **secret**?

4) Do you *want* to **share** your **secret** yet?

5) What are the *safe ways* to **tell him** your **secret?**

6) How do you *stay in your power* when *sharing* your **secret,** regardless of the outcome?

Now, you are going to have access to the techniques I had to create over the years to help me successfully handle any intimate situation. With these useful tips, you will once again be able to enjoy beautiful romance without any emotional distractions or attachments.

Most of all, you can live through the hair loss experience without anyone discovering your secret – until you want them to know it. This is the key to *Sex, Wigs & Whispers*.

I'm not concerned about judgment because as you will soon see, I've become accustomed to it. There will be those who will judge just because they have nothing better to do. Others, who have never looked truthfully into their heart in such a way, experience discomfort at being 'in touch' to a deeper degree. They may ultimately find it more comfortable to stand back and look for the negatives. Either way, this is unimportant to me. The information and experiences in this book are real life.

Either you want to go there with me or you don't. You need to know that you will never be the same person you were after you have finished it.

We'll explore the different choices available in how to present the truth to your friends, employers and potential mates. Through much trial and tribulation, I have learned that the reaction you get from sharing your secret has much to do with the way you present it.

This book will give you a number of positive ways to receive your best response.

This "little lady" is for your enlightenment, to carry and support you. Now you'll never be without solutions, or feel out of control. You may never need some of these techniques, but for others... they'll be glad they had this to turn to!

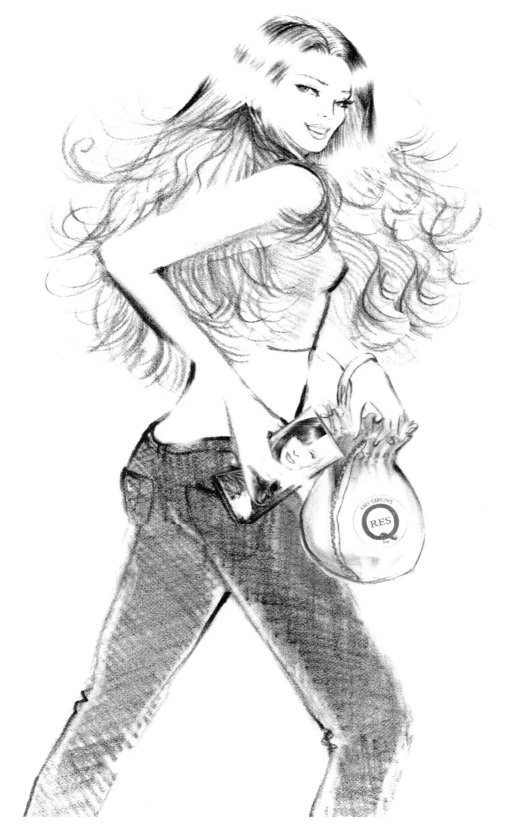

The History of Hair

Gimme a head with hair

Long beautiful hair

Shining, gleaming,

Streaming, flaxen, waxen

Give me down to there hair

Shoulder length or longer

Here baby, there mama

Everywhere daddy daddy

Hair, hair, hair, hair, hair, hair, hair

Flow it, show it

Long as God can grow it

My hair

Lyrics from the musical "Hair"

Why Are We So Caught Up About Our Hair?

There it was...the theme song of the late '60s...the follow up to when those four mop topped lads from Liverpool (The Beatles) burst onto the scene. Hair was the calling card of the era; a sign of protest and the signature of the day. From rallying against the war in Vietnam to Woodstock, hair – the longer the better – was the most visible symbol of it all.

But long before Camelot took over 1600 Pennsylvania Avenue, hair had a long history of its own.

So... how did the whole big deal about hair get started?

As we'll see in a Brief History of Hair, the meanings and importance of hair has permeated our societies and impacted us deeply, globally, for centuries:

Egypt:

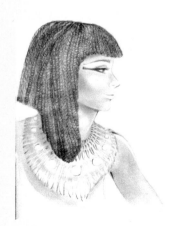

In the heat of Egypt, noblemen and women clipped their hair close to the head. But for ceremonial occasions heavy, curly black wigs were donned. Women's wigs were often long and braided, adorned with gold ornaments or ivory hairpins. Men's faces were generally clean shaved, but they sometimes wore stiff false beards.

Sex, Wigs and Whispers

GREECE:

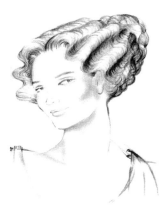

In classical Greece, women's hair was long and pulled back into a chignon. Many dyed their hair red with henna and sprinkled it with gold powder, often adorning it with fresh flowers or jeweled tiaras.

ROME:

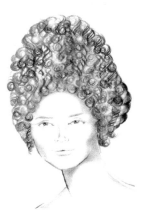

In austere Rome, the tendency was to follow Greek styles. The Roman upper classes would use curling irons and favored the gold powdered look of the Greeks. Women often dyed their hair blonde or wore wigs made from hair of captive civilization and slaves. Later, hairstyles became more ornate with hair curled tight and piled high on the head often shaped around wire frames. Hairdressing became popular and the upper classes were attended to by slaves or visited public barber shops.

China:

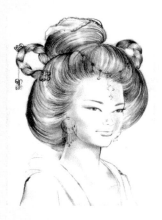

Unmarried Chinese girls' hair was usually worn long and braided while women combed the hair back from the face and wound into a knot at the nape.

Japan:

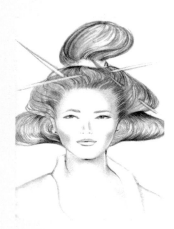

During the Medieval period, women's hair had been long and loose, but by the 17th century the hair became more styled, swept up from the nape of the neck and adorned with pins and jeweled combs. Geisha women's hairdos were especially elaborate, high and heavily lacquered and often enhanced with hairpieces.

Sex, Wigs and Whispers

AFRICA:

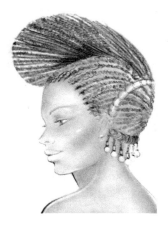

Due to the many tribal customs, African hairstyles were many and varied and usually signified status. Masai warriors tied the front hair into sections of tiny braids while the back hair was allowed to grow to waist length. Non-warriors and women however, shaved their heads. Many tribes dyed the hair with red earth and grease – some even stiffened it with animal dung. The complex style of the Mangbetu women involved plaiting the hair thinly and arranging over a cone-shaped basket frame, flaring the top then adorning the whole thing with long bone needles. Other tribes such as the Miango took a more simple approach, covering their long ponytails with a headscarf and adorning with leaves.

RENAISSANCE:

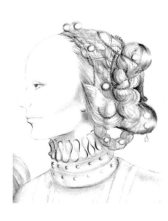

In the 1400s during the Renaissance, the ladies of the upper classes really took 'plucking' to its limit! If you think tweezing the odd eyebrow here and there is painful, imagine yourself plucking the entire front hairline away to give the appearance of a higher forehead! The rest of the hair was tightly scraped back to show off the elaborate headdresses of the day.

This was a practice common in Europe although the upper class ladies of Italy preferred to cover the hairline with low caps and jeweled turbans. They did, however, envy the fairer hair of Northern Europeans and sat for many hours in the heat of the sun in an attempt to bleach their hair (sound familiar?). The 'bleach' of the day was made using either saffron or onion skins.

Native American Indians:

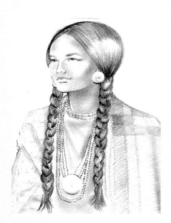

Native American Indians were divided in their hairstyles – those on the American East Coast sported entirely shaved heads, except for a ridge of hair along the crown; while Plains Indians, both men and women, wore the recognized long braids adorned with feathers. Further South, the Incas sported black headbands over relatively short often bobbed hair, while Aztec women plaited their hair entwined with strips of colored cloth then wound around the head. The Mayan nobility, although having shaved heads, donned high, ornate headdresses.

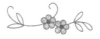

By the end of the 1500s in England, the hairstyles of the middle and upper classes had become quite elaborate. Led by their fashion-conscious queen, the ladies of England padded, curled, dyed, and ornamented their hair. Though blonde was the fashionable color for other countries (Sound familiar? Over

Sex, Wigs and Whispers

the last decade, more hair dyes are in blonde shades than any other), the English women of the era were loyal to Elizabeth and flame-red hair was the most popular color for women. The unreliability and harshness of hair dyes (most were extremely poisonous) also meant that there was a thriving business in wigs and hair pieces for women unsatisfied with their own hair (this is in the 16th Century! Wigs are big!).

As Queen Elizabeth's influence waned at the end of the 1500s, new technology appeared on the horizon (including the invention of the hair crimp) which enabled women to create a variety of styles that were previously unknown to them. These high-feathered hairstyles had universal appeal and swept throughout the entire European continent.

However, by the end of the 1600s, stacking rather than curling the hair was in vogue; often ornamenting the style with a bonnet or hat.

The Victorian Era, a generally repressed period all around, began when Queen Victoria was crowned in 1837 and lasted until her death in 1901. In the early part of her reign, the majority of women had very smooth, rigidly center-parted hair which was tightly pulled back and pinned into a bun. With the introduction of the heated curling iron in 1872, women began to curl their hair before braiding it and pinning it up into a bun.

And hair has had a central place in Fairy Tales and Mythology as we see with our dear Rapunzel and Lady Godiva (I'm leaving out the Biblical reference to Sampson's hair, but that was about the power of hair also – why did he become weak when it was cut off?).

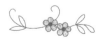

RAPUNZEL:

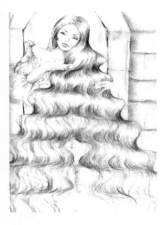

The famous children's writers, the Brothers Grimm, wrote specifically about the significance of hair in one of their most famous and beloved stories of all time: Rapunzel. The tale of "the most beautiful child in the world with long golden hair", who was being kept 'safe' in a tower by an evil witch with no way to leave. When Rapunzel tells the witch about a handsome Prince she's met (who climbs up her hair to visit with her!), the witch cuts off her hair; when the Prince finds Rapunzel without her long hair his touch causes her hair to regrow. This is a hairy story with deep implications.

LADY GODIVA:

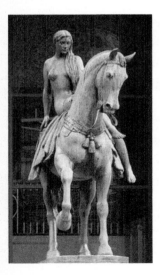

The legend of Lady Godiva, who rode naked through the streets of Coventry with only her long hair to cover her as a cloak in order to gain remission of the oppressive taxation imposed by her husband on his tenants. The one person in town, who looked at her against orders, became known as "Peeping Tom." Was it the nakedness or the hair that was of greatest importance?

So as you can see, for hundreds of years, hair has represented tremendous power and great significance – for reasons that go beyond fashion into politics, royalty, tradition and status.

Hair transmits a sense of self-expression, position and cultural conditions. And the times... have not changed.

And Ah, the 20th century... when women really started to come into their own. Driven by technological innovations, as well as changes in social norms, women began to move from the strictly domestic sphere to an active role in both professional and public life. And in the process, they bobbed their hair, rouged their knees, and learned the Charleston! The 1900s also bore witness to women in the war effort in the form of Rosie the Riveter in the 40s, the June Cleavers of the 50s, the Flower Children of the 60s referred to in the opening, and two television stars – Farrah Fawcett in the 70s and Jennifer Aniston in the 90s, who will long be remembered for their 'dos' when their acting roles for which they were created are long forgotten.

If you've ever wondered why at times hair has held such importance for you, it's partly not your fault. Think about the strong subliminal messaging there is around hair everywhere you turn and as far back as you can remember: Movies, TV shows, Magazines, beauty ads, all the commercials with all the girls swinging their gorgeous hair in the wind...

And then... there's Barbie Doll.

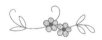

BARBIE

"My whole philosophy of Barbie was that through the doll, the little girl could be anything she wanted to be. Barbie always represented the fact that a woman has choices."

Ruth Handler (creator of the Barbie doll), on being inspired by her young daughter Barbara's fascination with teenage life and love for fashion dolls.

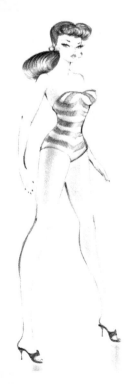

Barbie Millicent Roberts (the Barbie Doll), made her first appearance in public on March 9, 1959 at the New York Toy Fair. Her first look was intended to mirror the sophisticated glamour of 1950s stars like Marilyn Monroe and Rita Hayworth: high arched brows, pursed red lips, a sassy pony tail with curly bangs and a coy, sideways glance.

Barbie has continued to evolve in many ways. She was, and still is, the most iconic figure for little girls who dream glamorous dreams about being beautiful and having beautiful hair to go with it. Sounding familiar?

Sex, Wigs and Whispers

However, before we can make positive changes in how we handle the emotions attached to our hair, we must first become aware of those things that have kept us attached to those emotions. Then, we can make the shifts necessary to get beyond what has been holding us back from what's truly important: self-confidence, gratitude, kindness, joy and love.

Awareness is the key – and always the first step.

Now that you realize more about how hair has found its place into your unconscious (and your salon bills), you are ready to better take in the messages I'm hoping to communicate in **Sex, Wigs & Whispers**, and let go of some of what's been holding you back to create the life you want to have - hair or no hair.

This book is not about your hair – or your baldness; it's about your inner essence and power and reconnecting with what lights you up.

You *can* learn when to claim these qualities, when to hold on to them and when to share them – as your own choice. Indeed, you must learn to make these choices, for your own inner beauty.

No one knows better than you the limitations you have placed on yourself; it takes waking up and courage to be creative and move through them. Only you dream your dreams. There's nothing to stop you from living them.

PART

1

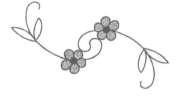

My Story

Growing Up

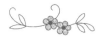

Life is not what it's supposed to be.
It's what it is.
The way you cope with it is what
makes the difference.

Virginia Satir

AT AN EARLY AGE I KNEW I WAS DIFFERENT...

LITTLE DID I KNOW WHAT THAT REALLY MEANT.

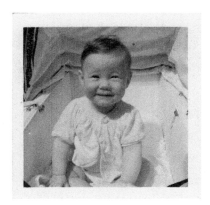

I was born into a creative, colorful and dynamic, upper middle-class family in Westchester, New York. My mother was a talented fashion designer; my father – a women's ready-to-wear buyer and retailer, former landscape architect and singer on early 1940's radio. My sister followed in his footsteps, aspiring to be the next big pop star.

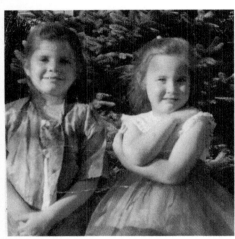

JODY AND I

My parents met when my father came in to purchase new styles for his stores from the manufacturer my Mom designed for. He was innovative and one step ahead when it came to women's fashions. I heard stories of other retail buyers waiting until my dad would leave a buying office or manufacturer to find out what 'Bobby bought today,' as most of his picks were right on the money.

They say opposites attract and such was the case with my parents; Dad was a loner and not very social. Mom was outgoing; a total 'people person' with a quick wit, great sense of humor, ballsy and fun. This was showcased most in her presentation splendor when entertaining small and large groups. She loved sunbathing and hanging with her girlfriends around the incredible landscape my father had created; a huge roman shaped pool

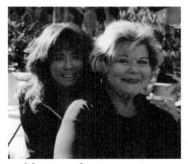

MOM AND I AT A SMASHING JULY 4TH PARTY IN LOS ANGELES

Sex, Wigs and Whispers

surrounded by a perfect bed of roses, a colorful cabana with a bar that was always kept fully stocked and a man-made stone wall surrounding it all – encasing it in its beauty of an array of natural colors. It was absolutely magnificent.

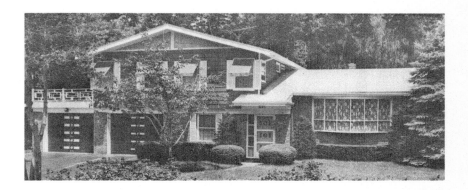

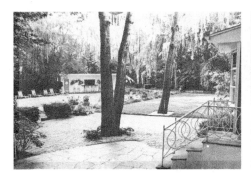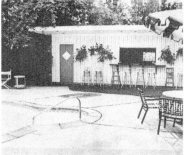

OUR HOME

For five hours every other Monday, my mother hosted bridge with her friends. She kept two meat freezers and a huge refrigerator packed to the rim; something I still consider a necessity of life. *LOL*

Oy – and I wonder where my food addiction comes from?!

Food shopping was never an errand, but a reverent activity. I am like my mother in all things food and entertaining.

Growing Up

Sunday mornings were filled with my Mom and I, soaking in volumes of Dr. Barker's spiritual lectures on the Science of Mind[1], along with Edgar Cayce, an American psychic best known for his predictions. Cayce was fascinating, and with only a ninth grade education, managed to possess this ability to heal patients while in a trance. I remain intrigued.

My father's eavesdropping would find him confused, bewildered or sometimes in judgment about what the hell we were listening to. Mom and I chuckled. A few times we felt both frustrated and almost disgusted by Dad's inability to be open – if only for a moment. But we quickly let go of that judgment and stayed focused on our precious time together. Spirituality bonded us. I remember at the tender age of seven when my Grandma Sarah, dad's mom, died; I said to mom,

"Why are you going to the funeral? Her spirit, which is the only thing that matters, is already gone. It's a waste of time and money."

My mother's jaw dropped. That moment cemented together, our unique spiritual beliefs. Nothing more needed to be said. Out of respect, we both went to the funeral together and observed this traditional rite of passage. It's been five years since my own mother's passing and I still speak and pray aloud to her every day.

At the age of seven and a half, Mom introduced me to 'private séances,' like the kind you see with a Ouija Board; only these were conducted by our neighbor, also a well-known psychic. In one of the more interesting sessions, titles like 'Love of Life,' 'Young and the Restless' and 'Airplane' were spelled out to me. We had no idea what those clues meant at the time, but as I would discover in acting roles years later, those show titles would echo in my ears, as I effortlessly landed parts in those shows, hands down.

· · · · · · · · · · · ·

1   Not to be confused with Scientology, as it's completely different.

Sex, Wigs and Whispers

Casting agents would say to Mom,

"My God, it's amazing how confident and relaxed your daughter was; she gave a great audition. It was as if she already knew she had the part."

My mom would turn and give me a little wink and we shared a silent chuckle.

I always wondered why my Mom married my father; she was so spiritual, while he was completely external, superficial and for the most part semi-conscious. At age 10, I questioned her about this and her reply is still vivid in my mind,

"Your father and I have karma, Honey; you know how that works."

And I did; so I never asked again. My dad had a generous heart and was a good provider when it came to our family's needs. This sense of security held great importance to her.

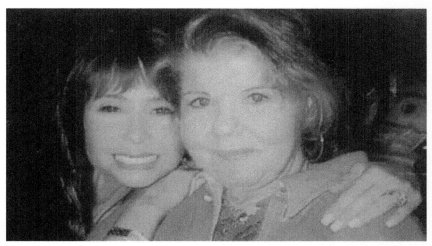

MOM AND I AT DINNER BEFORE, UNBEKNOWNST TO ANYONE, SHE HAD CONTRACTED CREUTZFELDT-JAKOB DISEASE. I LOST HER SO QUICKLY IN JUST 7 WEEKS AFTER HER ARRIVAL IN LOS ANGELES.

At 21, my father was 'discovered' while working as a pageboy for CBS Radio; when unbeknownst to him, the microphone was on as he was singing a song to himself and was accidentally overheard by a studio CEO. This led to starring roles on the first radio soap-opera *Big Sister,* with the big band impresario Guy Lombardo, among others. Somewhat overshadowed by his sister, the Platinum selling, #1 songstress from 1950's, also the personal choice of Grace Kelly at her wedding to Monaco's Prince Rainier, along with her very own star on Hollywood Boulevard, she was commonly referred to as *'Her Nibs-Georgia Gibbs'.* So music had a big influence in our home. I always gravitated to Barry Manilow, Barbara Streisand and anything Motown.

At the tender age of 8 months, something very traumatic would find me in the company of doctors and hospitals for quite some time; Mom was entertaining and a woman with the vicious virus staphylococcus on her hand had touched my bottom, leaving its infectious mark. This would have me struggling with pus, boils and this awful condition over the next five years. In the hope of finding a remedy for my suffering it seemed there were only two treatments that existed at that time:

1) Tetracycline, which turned my teeth brown.

2) Dipping me in extremely hot water, so that the toxic pus from the boils on my bottom would burst into the steaming water and prevent it from going back into my bloodstream.

TETRACYCLINE DAMAGE TO MY TEETH WERE OBVIOUS HERE

I vividly remember screaming from the pain as they quickly dipped me into the hot water over and over again. At age 5, it subsided, until I was 13, when it reared its ugly head again on the back of my knees, then disappeared again shortly thereafter.

Sex, Wigs and Whispers

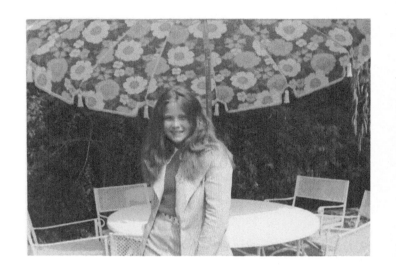

AGE 13

NOW YOU CAN
SEE WHY I WAS
SO ATTACHED TO
MY BEAUTIFUL MANE

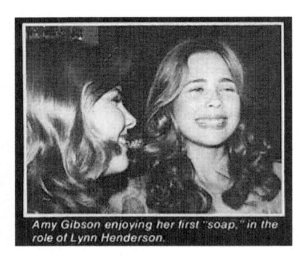

Amy Gibson enjoying her first "soap," in the role of Lynn Henderson.

My first interview after landing a leading role on "Love of Life" for CBS

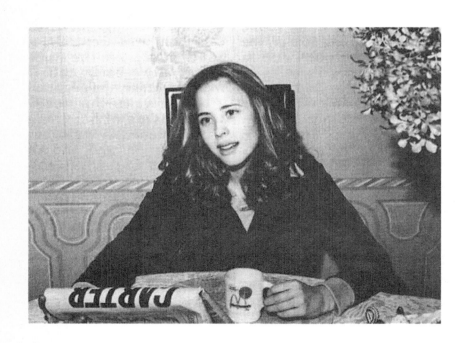

Sex, Wigs and Whispers

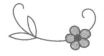

My First Interview

Prior to landing my first acting job on the soap opera *Love of Life*, my Mom and I decided it was best for me to fire my personal manager and have her take over and manage my career. Shortly after, one of my Mom's clients happened to bring her a charismatic young man from her acting class. He was good looking, smart and gave a great audition. Everything was a win-win except for his name: Tom Mapother the Third.

My Mom was preparing to go on vacation and travel magazines were spread out before her. She suddenly had a thought and looked at him intensely and said, "Oh, that name definitely won't work, you're going to be "Tom Cruise." She continued to work with Tom and many other wonderful actors and made quite a name for herself in the industry for over 20 years.

My next traumatic experience would find me only six months later while starring on my very first soap-opera, CBS's *Love of Life* during hair & makeup before a taping, I turned my head over to brush my hair, and received an earful from my hair stylist Nick, who informed me,

"Whoa Amy, did you know you have a bald spot the size of the palm of your hand?"

I thought he must be kidding. He then gave me a hand mirror and I was stunned. I mean, when do you really see your scalp? So, intrigued at first, I quickly turned to 'freaked-out' in seconds!

I must have associated this with a documentary on Leprosy, because I was suddenly worried about losing my limbs and skin too! I went into an emotional spin, crying hysterically. But then there was a sort of calm; like after one gets when hit with horrible news, followed by the numbness of shock. I did my scenes as if I were on auto-pilot and left as quickly as possible. The following day my Aunt Georgia took me to the leading dermatologist, since she knew every doctor in New York. He informed us that I had an immune disorder called Alopecia, and that there was no cure for this affliction to my hair and head, just what was considered a 'Band-Aid; treatment that consisted of shooting Triamcinolone, (a popular cortisone to this day used for re-growth) straight into my scalp near the bald spots. I thought, *You can't be serious!*

The train ride back to Westchester seemed to take twice as long. Between being consumed with everyone's hair and the loss of my own, and what had just transpired at the doctors, it was difficult to decipher my thoughts. On the way home from the train station my Mom and I discussed what was ahead for both of us and as usual, she found a way to try and turn it around to see the positive in this experience. But at that moment, it was near impossible for me to comprehend. When we walked into the house we found my father sitting in the corner of the living room and 'over the top' emotional. I immediately turned to my mother and said,

"Shouldn't that be me?"

In reading the following chapters, you will soon understand his response.

Cortisone injections often stimulate hair re-growth. Twenty to thirty injections, per patch, were required once a month.

Sex, Wigs and Whispers

The injections were very uncomfortable. Cortisone injections only work in the areas that have been injected; the injections do not prevent new areas of hair loss. It generally takes one to two months after the injections, before hair growth is visible. Some patients do not respond to any treatment. They cannot predict which patients will respond to treatment and which will not. Cortisone creams are also sometimes beneficial in the treatment of Alopecia Areata.[2] Hidden from the nurses, I would breathe in the freezing spray they used to numb my scalp before treatment. This would get me high enough to handle the cringe from the sound of Rice Krispies, as their huge needle entered deep and violated my scalp.

It was always a matter time before I would receive their famous words of wisdom; "Amy, if it's not broken why fix it. It's working Amy, that's all that counts at the moment until we learn more. At least be happy with that!"

As if they had any idea of what spending the rest of my life burdened with this uncertainty – would be like. On many occasions after listening to this, I would lose my temper from sheer frustration and storm out angrily crying, vowing to search for a new doctor who was more informed; someone out there, who could tell me something different for once; someone who would be able to give me ANY hope. After fruitless trips to London, France, Italy and Switzerland, with the best experts money could buy, I was still no closer to finding out how to tame this out-of-control animal. Regardless of the amount of doctors, specialists or healers I consulted, no one could assist me in dealing with this condition, either emotionally or physically. Clearly, it seemed No Real Answers existed.

. . . .

2   Alopecia Areata – a medical term meaning hair loss.

And since the government considered this condition to be an 'emotional disorder caused by stress' there was little funding for research or assistance for those in need. Although Alopecia is more commonly known today, research funds are still minimal. It's for this reason we are no closer to a cure and that so many people are still unaware of the condition and remain in a state of confusion and fear. Only recently have there been a couple of hopeful trials that are showing promise. However at $7000 a month, few people will be able to afford this treatment. Hopefully the pharmaceutical companies will make this treatment available at a cost that makes sense for so many in need.

Although the cortisone did create re-growth, this painful treatment was only temporary until the next month, when another bald spot would appear. These spots had begun to appear more frequently each time, coming in larger than the month before. I couldn't think too far ahead, and never knew what I was going to be faced with next.

My sister was always very supportive trying to do her best to convince me that it wasn't that bad. But I just couldn't go there with her. There was too much fear, and such a heavy sense of loss that could not be communicated to anyone at that time. So most of the time, I would shove the grief as far down as it would go; trying to move forward with what was in front of me. I would simply tell myself, *"I'll deal with 'this' later."*

I found it most interesting that my mother never shed a tear with me over my hair loss; at least not one that I could see. There were a couple of times I remember hearing her cry under the covers and asking God *"why?"*

As so many women feel about their children who are stricken with hair loss, she too felt that it was due to the extra glass of wine she may have had while pregnant. Most men carry the guilt of it having something to do with their sperm. Neither are true nor have any bearing on hair loss. Much of the time, Alopecia is unexplainable. But Mom was always wearing a brave face. What an amazing force of nature she was! She couldn't wait for me to write this book! This gives me peace because I feel her here with me and so present as I write this.

I knew my time in New York was finished and it was time to head to Los Angeles to fulfill my dreams of taking on challenging roles and emulating the career of "Sally Field", whom after seeing Sybil, I had great respect for. I had been counting down the days for months and preparing to go, silently journaling every day.

One day my Mom came over for an impromptu visit and said,

"So Am, let me ask you something? If you're going to Hollywood like you say for Pilot season only, which you know only lasts three to four months, then why did you pack your dishes?"

I hadn't even realized I did this. Then again, I was totally ready for my next adventure and wasn't surprised.

So off I went.

After working on Love of Life for 3 years and putting in many long hours on print and modeling jobs, television commercials and voice overs, and literally working my butt off for so many years, you would think I would have ended up with quite a nest egg. At least that's what I had planned for. However unfortunately when I arrived in Los Angeles expecting to only focus on my career and acting classes, I came to find out that the manager my parents had entrusted all my funds to ended up squandering all but $3500 dollars of my entire savings on dry oil wells, leaving me to suddenly live out of a 400 square foot studio apartment with a warming plate, a Murphy bed that came out from the wall like in *"I Love Lucy"* and driving a beat up Datsun with a missing back window, instead of my beautiful home and Mercedes that I had worked towards and dreamed of for years.

The only girl I knew in Los Angeles was the daughter of a famous actor with whom I had worked in New York. Where I expected her to keep her promise of helping me acclimate to Los Angeles and introduce me to people, she was so intimated she never took me anywhere nor did she introduce me to one person. I was on my own from the get go.

There I was at seventeen and a half, trying to figure it out and feeling so alone, angry, and disappointed. Yet I had such an incredible drive to succeed here, regardless of circumstances, that it was the only thing I focused on and everything else seemed to fall to the wayside.

To make ends meet, I worked three waitressing jobs a day; the early breakfast shift at a deli from 5:30 AM-10 AM, then would hop over to another restaurant to serve the lunch crowd from 11:30-3PM, take auditions whenever possible, then go home and rest before leaving for my nighttime job at The Daisy, a top Beverly Hills club where I would then serve the VIP's of Hollywood. It certainly gave me an interesting perspective to say the least.

One of my waitressing highlights was when I lied to get a job at a French restaurant where Caesar salads were made fresh at each table. On my first night, one of my dinner guests looked up at me and said,

"Wow, aren't you Lynn Henderson from Love of life?" For which I quickly rambled,

"Yes, and tonight's special is Beef Bourguignon!"

Sex, Wigs and Whispers

For weeks I would peek at the cook book beneath the napkin under my chef table until I got the hang of it. I worked there for a few months until one evening a dashing couple came in both dressed in monochromatic creme microsuede suits. Throughout the evening her husband kept making advances toward me. Careful not to endanger my tip I purposely directed all my attention towards her, which is why I was surprised at that happened next. As I went to reach to empty her cigarette butts from the ashtray, she seemed to conveniently miss the ashtray and instead put her cigarette out on my hand. I couldn't believe her phony reply,

"Oh, I'm sooo sorry".

Well, needless to say when it was time for me to serve their whipped cappuccino and I just 'happen' to trip causing the coffee to splatter all over their designer suits, I was sure to give her the same response. Of course, you know what happened next. Yes, I was fired.

The competition in Hollywood is fierce so you've got to be at the top of your game to the best of your ability. There is the tremendous financial commitment most actors need to make for their career prior to making it big that people rarely hear about. Aside from the normal overhead rent – food, gas, etc., are expensive photo shoots, acting, dance, and exercise classes. Since my parents were able to only help me with a small portion of these expenses I lived the typical actress life; waitressing, working as a personal assistant and doing temp jobs, *which were always interesting as I was technically challenged to say the least.* I took whatever job came up to help me afford all that was needed.

My mission was clear and nothing was going to stop me from my goals of great success. In my mind if I had to work 3 jobs to get by, so be it!

I'll never forget when I lied to get an interview with the wife of a big producer and boasted about my organizational and computer skills. We were getting along great and all was going perfectly until... she asked me to work her computer and I couldn't find the power button!

There are many humorous waitressing stories as people are never more ornery then when their hungry, but for now let's stay on point.

After many auditions and studio screen tests, always coming soo close but never nailing it, I finally got a break with a small part in the movie "Airplane". *That's right, remember the words that were spelled out in the seance I spoke of earlier . . .*

It would take three more years of odd jobs, commercials and radio voice overs before I would land a wonderful role on "Young and The Restless" which lasted three years opposite Phil Morris, son of Gregg Morris from **Mission Impossible.**

I was careful to stay current with my Cortisone treatment and it served me well. However, you could definitely see where my hair had thinned from when I first began the show. The hair stylists would comment from time to time, and I would make up an excuse that I was on going though a thyroid issue which made sense as my weight always fluctuated. Hair spray and mousse helped keep it looking thick so I was able to protect my secret.

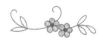

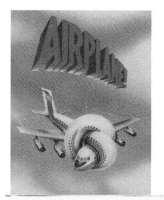

MAN FROM INDIA.........................JESSE EMMETT
FIRST JIVE DUDE...........NORMAN ALEXANDER GIBBS
SOLDIER'S GIRL...............................AMY GIBSON
MRS. GELINE........................MARCY GOLDMAN
STRIPED CONTROLLER...............BOBBY GORMAN
JOEY.....................................ROSSIE HARRIS
REPORTER #3........................MAURICE HILL

THE CAST

KAREEM ABDUL-JABBAR
AS MURDOCK
LLOYD BRIDGES
AS McCROSKEY
PETER GRAVES
AS CAPTAIN OVEUR
JULIE HAGERTY
AS ELAINE
ROBERT HAYS
AS TED STRIKER
LESLIE NIELSEN
AS DR. RUMACK
LORNA PATTERSON
AS RANDY
ROBERT STACK
AS KRAMER
STEPHEN STUCKER
AND INTRODUCING OTTO
AS HIMSELF

RELIGIOUS ZEALOT #6..........JIM ABRAHAMS
VICTOR BASTA...............FRANK ASHMORE
GUNDERSON.............JONATHAN BANKS
PAUL CAREY.............CRAIG BERENSON

JIVE LADY...................BARBARA BILLINGSLEY
MRS. HAMMEN.................LEE BRYANT
MRS. DAVIS.................JOYCE BULIFANT
SECURITY LADY.............MAE E. CAMPBELL
AIRPORT STEWARD...............TED CHAPMAN
FIRST JIVE DUDE.....NORMAN ALEXANDER GIBBS
SOLDIER'S GIRL.................AMY GIBSON
MRS. GELINE................MARCY GOLDMAN
STRIPED CONTROLLER.........BOBBY GORMAN
JOEY........................ROSSIE HARRIS
YOUNG BOY WITH COFFEE.......DAVID HOLLANDER
JAPANESE GENERAL...........JAMES HONG
JACK......................HOWARD HONIG
RELIGIOUS ZEALOT #1.........GREGORY ITZIN
MAN IN TAXI................HOWARD JARVIS
NEWSCASTER.............MICHAEL LAURENCE
FIRST KRISHNA.............DAVID LEISURE
RELIGIOUS ZEALOT #2.........ZACHARY LEWIS
RELIGIOUS ZEALOT #3.......BARBARA MALLORY
NUN......................MAUREEN McGOVERN
COCAINE LADY..............NORA MEERBAUM
SHIRLEY...................MARY MERCIER
LIEUTENANT HURWITZ..........ETHEL MERMAN
REPORTER #1................LEN MOOY

HANDING LADY...............ANN M. NELSON
MRS. HURWITZ..............LAURA NIX
REPORTER #2................JOHN O'LEARY
SOLDIER.................CYRIL O'REILLY
HOSPITAL CONTORTIONIST.......BILL PORTER
MR. HAMMEN..............NICHOLAS PRYOR
RELIGIOUS ZEALOT #4......CONRAD E. PALMISANO
A. TICKET AGENT..........MALLORY SANDLER
YOUNG GIRL WITH COFFEE.....MICHELLE STACY
RELIGIOUS ZEALOT #5........ROBERT STARR
MRS. KRAMER.............BARBARA STUART
MRS. OVEUR................LEE TERRI
AIR CONTROLLER NEUBAUER.....KENNETH TOBEY
JACK KIRKPATRICK..........WILLIAM TREGOE
JAPANESE NEWSCASTER.........HATSUO UDA
AIR CONTROLLER MACIAS.......HERB VOLAND
WINDSHIELD WIPER MAN.......JIMMIE WALKER
LISA DAVIS................JILL WHELAN
SECOND JIVE DUDE...........AL WHITE
SECOND KRISHNA........JOHN-DAVID WILDER
HORSE.....................WINDY
DR. BRODY...............JASON WINGREEN
MRS. JAFFE................LOUISE YAFFE
MAKE-UP LADY............CHARLOTTE ZUCKER
GROUND CREWMAN #2..........DAVID ZUCKER
GROUND CREWMAN #1..........JERRY ZUCKER

TECHNICAL CREDITS

A HOWARD W. KOCH PRODUCTION
WRITTEN FOR THE SCREEN AND DIRECTED BY
JIM ABRAHAMS
DAVID ZUCKER
JERRY ZUCKER
PRODUCED BY.................JON DAVISON
DIRECTOR OF PHOTOGRAPHY....JOSEPH BIROC, A.S.C.
PRODUCTION DESIGNER.........WARD PRESTON
FILM EDITOR.............PATRICK KENNEDY
MUSIC BY.............ELMER BERNSTEIN
COSTUME DESIGNER.......ROSANNA NORTON
SET DECORATOR..........ANNE D. McCULLEY
EXECUTIVE PRODUCERS........JIM ABRAHAMS
DAVID ZUCKER
JERRY ZUCKER
ASSOCIATE PRODUCER..........HUNT LOWRY
SPECIAL THANKS TO...
KIM JORGENSEN
PAT PROFT

CASTING...................JOEL THURM
ADDITIONAL CASTING.........SUSAN ARNOLD
WALLY NICITA
GRETCHEN RENNELL
DIRECTOR OF PHOTOGRAPHY
SPECIAL EFFECTS...........BRUCE LOGAN
MINIATURE SPECIAL EFFECTS....RICHARD D. HELMER
SET DESIGNER...............JOE HUBBARD
MAKE-UP ARTIST........EDWIN BUTTERWORTH
HAIR STYLIST...............JOAN PHILLIPS
COSTUME SUPERVISOR..........AGGIE LYON
RECORDING MIXER...........TOM OVERTON
MUSIC EDITORS...........KATHY DURNING (LA DA
JEFF CARSON) PRODUCTIONS
SOUND EDITOR............JIM TROUTMAN
RE-RECORDING MIXERS......JOHN T. REITZ, C.A.S.
DAVID CAMPBELL
ROBERT PETTIS
UNIT PRODUCTION MANAGER....MAURICE VACCARINO
FIRST ASSISTANT DIRECTOR.......ARNIE SCHMIDT
SECOND ASSISTANT DIRECTOR.......KEN COLLINS
GAFFER...............LARRY GIL HOOLY
GRIPOLOGY............PETE PAPANICKOLAS
PROPERTY MASTER.........STEVEN LEVINE
SECRETARY TO MR. VACCARINO......BETTY MOOS

CAMERA OPERATOR.......FREDERICK J. SMITH
SPECIAL EFFECTS.........JOHN FRAZIER
GENERALLY IN CHARGE
OF A LOT OF THINGS.........MIKE FINNELL
AIRPORT ARRANGEMENTS......STEVE KRAMER
STUNT COORDINATOR....CONRAD E. PALMISANO
ASSISTANT CAMERA PERSONS.......TODD HENRY
JAMIE ANDERSON
ASSISTANT EDITOR...........SCOTT WALLACE
SCRIPT SUPERVISOR..........NANCY HANSEN
BOOM PERSON..............DENNIS JONES
CHOREOGRAPHER............TOM MAHONEY
MAGIC CONSULTANT........LARRY WILSON
DGA TRAINEE................DAN ATTIAS
PROCESS SUPERVISOR......DONALD HANSARD
EFFECTS UNIT GRIP..........JERRY DEATS
EFFECTS UNIT GAFFER.......BRINK BRYDON
ELECTRICAL DEPARTMENT......GARY WOSTACK
DANNY MARZOLD
GRIPS....................BILL DECKER
EDMOND WRIGHT
NICK PAPANICKOLAS
ASSISTANT PROPMASTER........TOM CROWL
COSTUMER...............VICTORIA SNOW
TRANSPORTATION............TOM BAKER
GLENDA BAKER
LEADPERSON.............MIKE HIGELMIRE
CONSTRUCTION COORDINATOR.....WALLY GRAHAM
STILLS...................JOHN MONTE
UNIT PUBLICIST............ART SARNO
WRANGLERS...............DICK WEBB
J.L. MITCHELL
CRAFT SERVICE.........ADAM CULLINGA
FIRST AID................DAVE MILLER
VOCAL EFFECTS ADVISOR.......ALLISON CAINE
AUTHOR OF "A TALE OF TWO CITIES"
CHARLES DICKENS
ORCHESTRATIONS............DAVID SPEAR
VISUAL EFFECTS BY:
MOTION PICTURE INCORPORATED/BLALACK & SHOURT
VISUAL CONCEPT ENGINEERING/PETER KURAN
MAGIC LANTERN/BILL HEDGE
SPECIAL PROJECTS/CHRIS WALAS
ROBERT KEITH & COMPANY, INC.

TITLE DESIGN/DAN PERRI
TITLES & OPTICALS BY JACK RABIN AND ASSOCIATES
ADDITIONAL OPTICALS—
HOWARD ANDERSON COMPANY
STAYIN' ALIVE
WRITTEN AND PERFORMED BY THE BEE GEES
COURTESY OF RSO RECORDS
PUBLISHED BY STIGWOOD MUSIC, INC.
THEME FROM "JAWS"
BY JOHN WILLIAMS
NOTRE DAME VICTORY MARCH
BY MICHAEL J. SHEA, J.H. O'DONNELL & JOHN F. SHEA
RIVER OF JORDAN
BY PETER YARROW
EVERYTHING'S COMING UP ROSES
BY STEPHEN SONDHEIM AND JULE STYNE
RESPECT
BY OTIS REDDING
THE PRODUCERS GRATEFULLY ACKNOWLEDGE:
TRANS AMERICAN FREIGHT LINES
ATARI, INC.
SCHUMACHER ANIMAL RENTALS
ARGON OIL COMPANY
RON SMITH LOOK-ALIKES
DICK LOWRY
LAURIE ABDO
SHERI MARUNO
PAUL TURNER
NANCY COCUZZO
DANICE HERTZ
DENNIS PARK
SHEILA SULLIVAN
TERRY SHADIN
ROBERT REILLY
RICHARD RAYNIS
SUSAN BRESLAU
JASON BLACK
ERIKA HILLER
CHRIS ROSS
CHRIS CASSIDY
PETER IVERS
KAREN RASCH

LENSES AND PANAFLEX CAMERA BY PANAVISION®
METROCOLOR®
MPAA SEAL AND CERTIFICATE NUMBER 25740
GLEN-GLENN SOUND
THE PERSONS AND EVENTS IN THIS FILM ARE FICTITIOUS. ANY SIMILARITY TO ACTUAL PERSONS OR EVENTS IS UNINTENTIONAL.
THIS MOTION PICTURE IS PROTECTED UNDER THE LAWS OF THE UNITED STATES AND OTHER COUNTRIES. UNAUTHORIZED
DUPLICATION, DISTRIBUTION, OR EXHIBITION MAY RESULT IN CIVIL LIABILITY AND CRIMINAL PROSECUTION.
A PARAMOUNT PICTURE
MPAA RATING: PG
MAIN & END TITLE BILLING
AS OF 5/2/80
© MCMLXXX PARAMOUNT PICTURES CORPORATION
ALL RIGHTS RESERVED

PG PARENTAL GUIDANCE SUGGESTED
SOME MATERIAL MAY NOT BE SUITABLE FOR CHILDREN

Growing Up

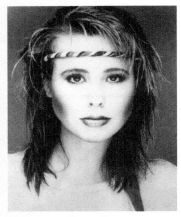

AGE 19 – FIRST HOLLYWOOD
PHOTO SHOOT

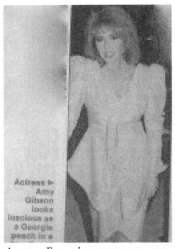

Actress
Amy
Gibson
looks
luscious as
a Georgia
peach in a

AT THE EMMY'S AFTER LANDING
THE ROLE ON Y&R

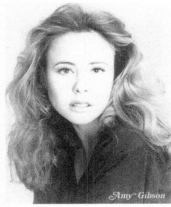

Amy Gibson

AGE 22 – COMING INTO MY OWN

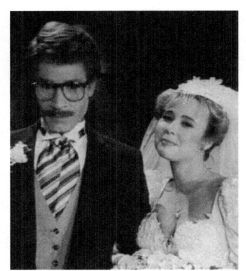

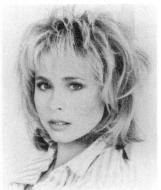

AUDITION PHOTOS FOR THE
ROLE OF 23 YEAR OLD VIRGIN
ALANA ANTHONY ON
YOUNG AND THE RESTLESS

MY Y&R CO-STAR; THE WONDERFUL AND
TALENTED PHIL MORRIS SPENT 3 HOURS A DAY
HAVING MAKEUP APPLIED TO ACHIEVE THE
LOOK OF A WHITE MAN FOR
THE ROLE OF TYRONE.

Sex, Wigs and Whispers

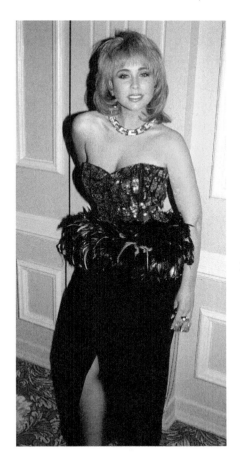

AT THE EMMY AWARDS
I LOVED THIS
OSCAR DE LA RENTA GOWN.
I STILL HAD MY HAIR
ALTHOUGH IT WAS THINNING.
PRODUCT HELPED IT LOOK FULLER,

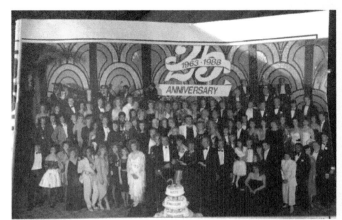

Y&R 20TH
ANNIVERSARY
CAST PHOTO.

Growing Up

I was grateful that for 17 years the cortisone shots kept my hair growing back and my secret quiet – until my bald spots became so prevalent that the cortisone became too much for my body to handle and I had to stop the shots. Regretfully, this was the only known treatment. It took just three weeks for me to lose all my hair and I was completely bald! This happened just five weeks before beginning a new show, and my most challenging role as an actress on *General Hospital*.

"What was I supposed to do, now?! My life is over!"

I suddenly found myself in the midst of a mini nervous breakdown.

However painful and frightening my hair loss roller coaster ride had been up to that point – a whole different journey began the day I actually lost all of my hair – every strand, every bit.

I could no longer cover up my hair loss by simply parting my hair differently or by just popping on a hat as if I were having a 'bad hair day.' Emotional pain, fear and lack of self-confidence redefined me. For the moment, I felt like I had lost all control over my life, had lost all of my power. I had no other option but to wear a full wig.

"What? I'm only 29 years old?!"

I felt stripped of my sexuality and femininity. I was angry with everyone – especially God. I would turn to the sky and desperately scream at the top of my lungs,

"Why did you do this to me! What do you want from me?"

Note: I've since come to find out that this is an understandable and a normal response. There is a grieving time that a person goes through when they have lost their hair (or what I sometimes refer to as, 'when your hair has chosen to leave'). It's important to honor these feelings and give yourself this time to move through

Sex, Wigs and Whispers

this process before you can find your essence again. I go into this in more detail later in the book.

I needed the acting job with *General Hospital* for the funds and for the advantage this opportunity afforded me in my career. It took several days for me to calm down and get a grip on my emotions.

Then, forced to conceal my terrible secret, I had to squelch my fear, summon up enough courage and try to quietly talk the producer into agreeing to turn my character into someone with several different looks and dialects to 'get her man'- thus allowing me to utilize wigs. Necessity is the Mother of invention! Equally important, I had to keep complete discretion from the network and the press. So, taking a deep breath, I met Wes, my producer, at a very public Beverly Hills coffee shop. I was confident that no matter what – I would not lose it there and thus be forced to keep it together. Wes and I had a professional history and he had always been loving and kind; available and willing to hear my creative thoughts, without judgments. This was so much more refreshing and inspiring than my father's continuous ridicule.

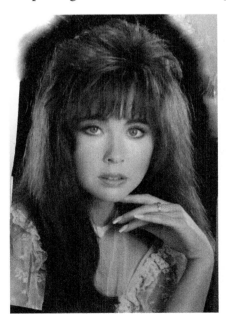

My first wig. I loved the color... but so much hair!

That day, I wore a red-colored wig under a hat. In retrospect, it's hard to believe with the amount of hair that was in that piece, that Wes didn't recognize its obvious added thickness, noticing it was a wig. But as you'll learn later in this book, men are often blind when it comes to wigs and hair. This experience with Wes was just another example.

After a few moments of chit chat, I broached the brilliant idea of turning my undercover agent character into someone who used several different looks, to get her man. When he took a beat before responding, I was certain he could hear my heart pounding. It was after all, my one and only brilliant idea in that moment; to which he replied,

"Wow, I love it! How interesting. I think the network will go for it; no one has ever done this before in daytime. How the hell did you come up with that?"

Taking a breath, I responded, *"Funny you should ask!"*

I took in another deep breath, and with all my might held back every tear of emotion I could, (which men don't respond well to anyway) and proceeded to tell him everything. When I was done, he sat there for a moment and said, "My God Amy, I am so sorry. You have really been through a lot. Ok, I think we can make this work. But, you have one hell of an acting challenge. I'll make sure no one finds out. Not even makeup or hair will ever say one word or they'll never work in this industry again! This will be our secret. But you have got to promise me to nail this role."

And I did just that.

In fact, years later, in 2006 when **People** magazine highlighted my **First Women's Swim Wig** design and the work I do with women and children, they questioned my producer Wes personally, asking if there had ever been any mention of a word about my hair to the press or the network. Wes kept his promise to me and never mentioned a single word about my missing hair, for which I am eternally grateful. (Thank you, Dear Wes.) And boy did he make it work! The wig disguises were marvelous, ranging from a short 'butch' blonde Russian, to a hardass redhead spy. My entrée into the world of wigs had begun. A hidden challenge however, was the fact that I had to make sure I wore the same wig to and from work every day to avoid any suspicion. And because my condition required complete and utter secrecy, I learned to lie extremely well to my cast mates, my family and most of my friends.

Other challenges would find me making excuses for a lack of personal appearances at celebrity sports events. The anticipation and fear of trying to potentially overcome something as simple as the wind blowing my hair away from my head and exposing my wig – would have left me humiliated, so I refused to attend. It became exhausting to constantly find ways to stop people from touching my hair or hugging me too hard for fear of my hair being pulled off (*another spontaneous fib: "Oh! Careful! Don't hug too hard! My neck is really out!"*) People would immediately retreat. This worked every time.

I was forced to deliver explanations to my PR people as to why, if I am such an amazing golfer, am I not taking part in all the celebrity golf tournaments being offered to me which would enhance my career. I would tell them, *"Oh I wish I could but I'm out of town that weekend at a personal growth seminar,"* or *"I tweaked my back and need to rest it for a bit",* or *"I wish I could I'm just really busy with so much work at the moment I just don't have the time right now."* Trying to remember what story I told to whom became an incredible challenge.

There is a big difference between being on a show where the perfect wigs are paid for and made to my specifications; with only the highest quality hair consistently maintained by my personal wig maker – and doing it all *myself.* The network accepted the change in my character on the show and put some of it in the budget; but in lieu of privacy and budget, I ultimately handled everything to do with *my wigs.* While at the same time, I was still trying to figure out how to survive with this foreign 'thing' on my head, nail my acting scenes and being totally 'normal' when I wasn't in front of the camera; and all of this without going broke.

I cried every night. Every morning I woke up exhausted and bewildered, scared of what the day would bring! I decided that I had no choice but to force myself the hell out of bed and 'go for it.' I would inspire myself by saying things like, *"Okay, it's time for battle!"*

I'd breathe through my moment of anxiety, move forward, and go.

I took many things for granted when I had hair, that I was suddenly faced with during my hair loss; like walking on the beach against the wind or opening a restaurant door while desperately trying to act nonchalant holding my 'new hair' in place. A quagmire of decisions appeared before me. I longed to be like every other woman, but I felt so different; weird, ugly, phony. I felt stripped of my former beauty. Seeing a woman with the hair I used to have would make me sick to my stomach. I'd catch myself staring at her long, beautiful hair.

The absence of any guidance to help me figure out who I was (or had become) as a bald woman was debilitating. There was no one to show me *how* to find a wig in the correct style and color. No one could show me *how* to *care* for these pieces or *how* to *wear* them in a way that would allow me to keep my secret safe.

Sex, Wigs and Whispers

Hiding my condition became fueled and driven by my fears. I had no idea how to share my secret with someone, even if I wanted to. There was no one to advise me and no manual; no idea how to tell my potential partner about my condition (or not), no idea how to keep anyone from finding out about my secret. There was no one to show me how to date with a wig on or how to live a normal life like any other woman; dancing, doing water sports, having wonderful relationships and being intimate. There was no guidance, no path; no one to advise me on how to deal with my partner discovering my private secret; I so wanted to just feel sensual without compromising my sexuality.

Am I ringing a bell here?!

My biggest issue was keeping myself feeling and looking like the woman I always was. At times, even that memory was difficult to find. I had to look at photos to remind myself, but then seeing my 'old-self filled me with sadness and rage, which only added to my depression.

Sound familiar?

Yet, I wasn't willing to just live in hiding and give up – nor should you. For my survival, I had to create subtle but useful techniques to help me get through my dating / life adventures. Little did I know, almost twenty years later, that so many women around the world would share these same techniques. So let's get to the big questions: the ones I had, and so many other women like you have…

How do you date successfully?

How do you have sex and enjoy intimacy with your wig on – without your partner ever finding out?

Growing Up

You'll soon learn that this is not a one-line answer, as there are many different scenarios covered in this book. However it's easier than you imagine.

If you can tap into these you'll do fine.

I'VE BEEN THERE – I'M STILL THERE. I GET IT! –

Okay, here we go!

AFFIRMATION

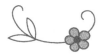

I am not swayed by appearances as I know they are not the 'truth'. The truth is, I am in total control of my choices and have the supreme ability to turn any situation around and manifest what I desire in my life.

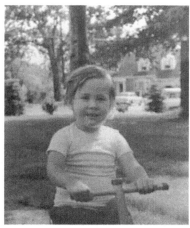

AGE 3 – ALWAYS SEEKING AN
ADVENTURE

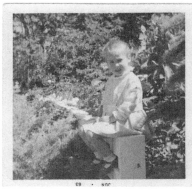

AGE 4 – JUST AFTER GETTING
CAUGHT REMOVING THE BUDS FROM
MY FATHER'S PRIZE WINING ROSE
COLLECTION.

I STILL LOVE THE FEEL OF ROSE PETALS

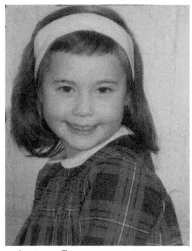

AGE 5 – CAN YOU BELIEVE HOW
SHORT THESE BANGS ARE?

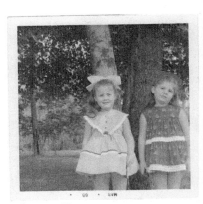

AGE 7 – TOBE JUST LOVED THOSE
BOWS!

Growing Up

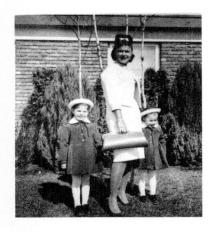

Being a designer, Tobe
definitely had her own style
and she made sure her girls
always followed in her foot
steps. I rarely remember a time
when my sister and I did not
wear matching outfits :)

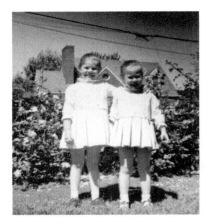

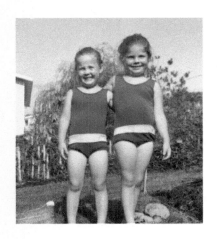

Sex, Wigs and Whispers

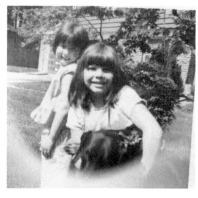

I THINK TOBE WAS IN A CREATIVE
MOOD ONE DAY AND PUT A BOWL
OVER OUR HEADS, TOOK A PAIR OF
SCISSORS AND JUST WENT TO TOWN!
ALTHOUGH TO MY SURPRISE WE
RECEIVED MANY COMPLIMENTS,
HYSTERICAL!

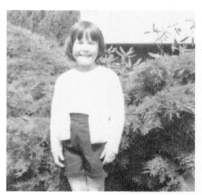

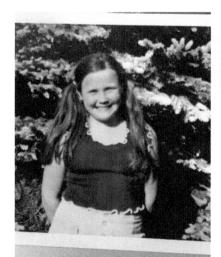

I WAS REALLY INTO MY PASTA.
DEFINITELY BEGINNING
MY PUDGY STAGE

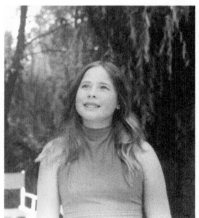

AT 12 3/4 YEARS – RIGHT BEFORE MY
BALD SPOTS STARTED

Growing Up

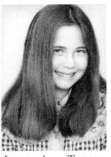

AGE 9 1/2 – TAKEN
AFTER CLASS AT
THE AMERICAN
ACADEMY OF
DRAMATIC ARTS

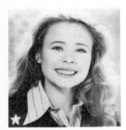

AGE 17 – THE
"ALL AMERICAN"
COMMERCIAL SHOT

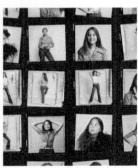

MY FIRST PROOF SHEET

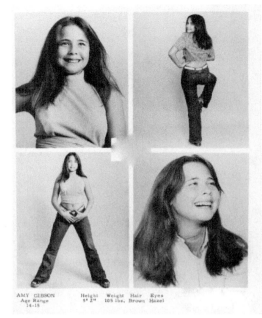

AMY GIBSON   Height Weight   Hair   Eyes
Age Range   5' 2" 105 lbs. Brown Hazel
14-15

MY FIRST PROFESSIONAL PORTFOLIO SHOTS

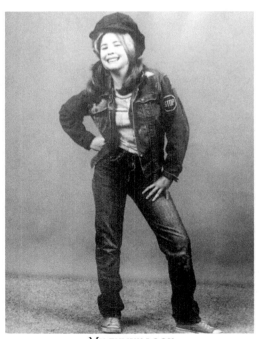

MY FUNKY LOOK

Sex, Wigs and Whispers

Since growing up with dachshunds, I've always had an affinity for those little hot dog dogs and have had many! They are such characters; extremely smart – hysterically funny but .. sooo defiant! If you have one, then you know exactly what I'm talking about.

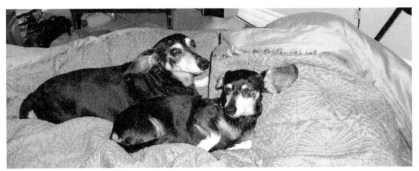

Harry The Hefty Handsome Hot Dog Dog and his beautiful wife Hanna filled my heart for well over a decade. It took years to recover after it was their time to leave me. Until recently when we got Punum; my Red Longhair Miniature Doxi who is undeniably the most loving, most beautiful Doxi I've ever experienced, and who like many Miniatures... has the spirit of a great dane.

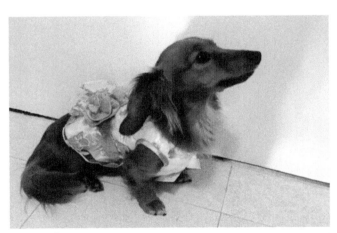

Okay – so I went a bit far here, but you have to admit she looks beautiful! Don't you just see her on the cover of "Iams" dog food?

Bill won't walk her if she's in any of her outfits. I told him that's ridiculous, she loooves to strut! (Still no luck!)

They truly are people with fur. We all hear of the animal abuse that takes place today in our country. How anyone could abuse these beautiful innocent beings is incomprehensible to me.

Growing Up

General Hell

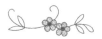

*"Nothing can dim the light which shines from within.
Courage is the most important of all the virtues
because without courage, you can't practice
any other virtue consistently."*

Maya Angelou

I never really got comfortable on General Hospital, commonly known as 'GH' in Hollywood. The experience on GH was agonizing because of the duration and the consistency of the terror I faced – or at least perceived that I faced – on a daily basis. My secret loomed over me every second of every day. There were numerous close calls and constant anxiety that my hidden truth would be exposed, like a black cloud over my head. The fear that I would be ousted from the show and the entire industry as a bald freak plagued me, leaving me in constant fear that I would lose everything and be left with nothing. I refer to this period of my life as 'General Hell' and at the same time, it was one of my greatest learning journeys.

After losing all my hair just five weeks prior to beginning my role on the show, I was recovering from a minor nervous breakdown while simultaneously taking on this challenging character and a brand new show. GH always had a reputation of being a difficult show and on-set environment for any new talent to break into. Clique doesn't even come close to what transpired on that set. Jealousy, insecurities and sometimes downright cruel behavior on the part of the actors on this show, are extremely difficult dynamics for anyone new to deal with; and to deal with it under these conditions, made the challenge even more arduous. My cast and crew didn't realize that for me, this was both a difficult new job and step in my career that I cared about; it was important to me, but also one of the most emotionally difficult times in my career *and* in my life. I came to understand that even if the cast had realized it, they couldn't have cared less.

There's no business like show business.

I rarely left my dressing room and cried most of the time counting down the weeks before my contract would end.

Each day was spent alone, constantly finding my way through a quagmire of confusion and fear about hiding my secret. There was no shared consideration or empathy. Adding to the stress was the emotional dysfunction of the set; mostly what I had to deal with from the other actors. Generally, actors can be cruel when they feel threatened. In all my years on television, the animosity I experienced came from the women, only on GH I had this experience with men as well. Eventually, I learned how to work around the backstabbing pettiness this particular group of actors seemed to exercise and enjoy. This group had been working together for over ten years and just did not accept anyone new. Their defensive and cloistered closed fraternity, was a soap opera sub-plot all its own that no one ever saw on air.

Regardless of the shallow and disturbing behavior that can exist, many wonderful actors do move on to stardom from soaps:

Alec Baldwin, *The Doctors*	1980-1982
Meg Ryan, *As the World Turns*	1982-1984
Marg Helgenberger, *Ryan's Hope*	1982-1986
Kyra Sedgwick, *Another World*	1982-
Demi Moore, *General Hospital*	1982 – 1983
Courteney Cox, *As the World Turns*	1984-
Robin Wright, *Santa Barbara*	1984-1988
Anne Heche, *Another World*	1988-1991
Ryan Phillippe, *One Life to Live*	1992 – 1993
Sarah Michelle Geller, *All My Children*	1993-1995
Paul Michael Glaser, *Love of Life*	1971
Dana Delany, *Love of Life*	1979-1980
Christopher Reeve, *Love of Life*	1974-1976
Eva Longoria, *The Young and the Restless*	2001 to 2003

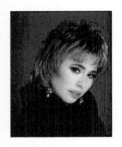

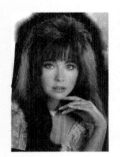

To make matters with my co-actors worse, I was given one of the major story lines of the summer – without a screen test or audition. This was viewed as my taking away time from their own storylines – stealing their 'moment'. What they didn't realize was that the part had been specifically created for me. Wes and I had worked together on *Young and The Restless*, and as he now moved on to produce *General Hospital* he created this role for me. The other actors assumed I was sleeping with him which was far from the truth. Wesley (Wes) was married and a dear friend and fan of my work. He wanted the ratings that a good storyline and actor could bring to the network; our last storyline that we had worked together on at CBS *Young and The Restless* was one of the first interracial storylines on daytime TV and had garnered several Emmy nominations. I needed the job, thrilled at the opportunity to step into such a fabulous character and to work on such a prestigious show. As I saw it, it was a win-win.

The way daytime soap operas work, there is a taping schedule and your scene is in a certain sequence. You arrive very early between 5-6 am for wardrobe, then onto makeup and hair. There are a variety of rehearsals throughout the day with your acting partners, all the while receiving notes from the producers, directors and/or writers prior to filming hours later. I arrived on my first day a bit nervous, keeping it together as best as I could under the circumstances. Per usual protocol, I was shown to my dressing room and given several pieces of clothing to try on for my upcoming scenes. Then I was off to the makeup room, where a lovely talented woman who I later learned was one of the best in the industry, greeted me. I took my seat and she began to work her magic. While in the midst of having only half my face finished, one of the actresses who had been on the show for years approached me and said, "Mmm... excuse me, but you're in my seat."

I had been warned about her attitude prior to joining the show from peers of mine who had worked with her. Not quite sure how to respond, but of course being a Sagittarius (Sagg's are best known for speaking honestly sans any diplomacy or tact, or maybe I just have a touch of Asperger's!), I spoke from the gut; without thinking first and certainly without editing, "Really, well I believe my scene precedes yours and so, instead of being rude to me on my first day, why don't you be a good little girl and take that seat over there. I'll let you know when I'm finished."

Wrong way to start this show.

She was very popular with the existing clique of actors so this only added fuel to an already well-built fire. I made it through the first day. That's the best thing I can say about it.

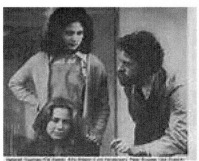

When I am alone, I take off my wig and put on a pretty turban. I do this for two reasons:

1) A common side effect of Alopecia is that I am always cold and the turban keeps my head warm.

2) It is important for me to feel good about how I look and do this for me. Turbans add color and a certain kind of energy, which is both feminine and uplifting. Of course putting on some gloss or lipstick always helps too!

General Hell

One day while in my dressing room preparing for a taping of one of the toughest scenes I had to do on GH, there was a knock on the door. I was in deep concentration on the sixty odd pages I had to memorize so I didn't hear it the first time; the next pounding got my attention. It was the director and he was obviously quite perturbed.

"Aaaammmmeeeey, are you in there? I need to see you immediately. There have been some last minute changes I need to go over with you, NOW! Get Out here!!!"

I freaked, grabbed my wig, and slopped it on my head! Between dealing with egos on a daily basis and hiding the truth, I had been walking on eggshells for months so I definitely didn't need this. I ran to the door so fast I forgot to look in the mirror! The minute I opened the door the frustration taking up most of his face was clearly intended for me and I got giddy. *Why giddy, you ask?* Unfortunately this is my normal response when I get nervous; which explains why I have always had a hard time at funerals or when someone gets upset with me. It's not that I am insensitive to the situation or the person; on the contrary, my entire life I've been faulted for feeling things too sensitively, as a result of being an actress. It's a knee-jerk reaction that occurs when I'm nervous and hard to control. It becomes a vicious cycle; I get nervous and start to laugh, then the other person gets angry thinking I am laughing *at* them, which of course makes me more nervous; thus, making me laugh even more and... so on. It calms down after I have had a chance to explain, which usually takes a few minutes. It usually works out, but sometimes not without drama.

The unannounced director looked at me rather strangely, took a beat, proceeded to give me my instructions and then abruptly left.

Sex, Wigs and Whispers

I was left there speechless. As I slowly turned to reenter my dressing room, I happened to catch my reflection in the mirror, and freaked! My wig was on backwards! That, at least in part, explains the expression on his face; I must have looked like 'Cousin It' from *The Adams Family.* My mind started to go in a thousand different directions. *Oh my god, he knows!* I was due on set and had to keep it together, at the same time feeling like a Rubik's cube in motion.

As with everything in the entertainment industry, it is better to play it cool and ignore a situation by pretending it never happened. So I did. However, this has always been a challenge, as I am the type of person who likes to get things clear as quickly as possible. Waiting for some time to pass, for things to calm down or sweeping something under the carpet is just not my style. I'm far more confrontational. It sometimes drives people crazy but *C`est la Vie.* This is who I am. I hate second guessing; too much work. I hate lying (anymore); too much to remember. A seeker of truth, my motto is 'Never ask me anything you don't want to know.'

In the land of Hollywood, you are taught early on that you never know where someone's professional position is going to be next, so never burn a bridge. After all, that assistant fetching your coffee could be the head of a network some day; so choose your battles carefully. Unfortunately, I've never been good at this because of too much ass-kissing. Way too phony. I refused to be pretentious, vying to remain true to myself and if doing this was going to hold me back from stardom and fame, then I chose not to have it at all.

It was finally time for me to come down for the taping of the show and the adrenalin in me was soaring. As I entered the sound stage I could hear the hustle-bustle taking place that I always loved before filming. There were lighting and cameramen checking their equipment, with stand-ins used to set up the shots. (A stand-in is a person with similar measurements to the star to stand in when the actor is unavailable.) There were actors running their scripts, while simultaneously having wardrobe and makeup working on last minute touch-ups; and the hyper director going over changes with the script supervisor assuring that everything is in order to begin filming. The whole scene is hectic, and intense – with a lot riding on each studio production, like everyone's jobs. As nervous as I was inside, whenever my back is up against the wall there is a survival side of me that always takes over in these situations. This comes from growing up in this business since the age of 9, and having to find ways to survive all the games that surround it. I cope by finding a deeper level of strength that mainly seems to surface in times like this.

I could see everyone scrambling in the corner of the stage. Between my earlier interaction with the director and shooting a tough scene, I was nervous because I had no idea what had really been seen during my wig catastrophe, and was scared and feeling extremely vulnerable. However, I couldn't, and wouldn't, let my fears about *him* throw me. I was determined to knock the socks off everyone in the control room; producer, network executive and everyone else on the set. I delivered and my performance was amazing. It was my way of showing the director I was not intimated by him.

It wouldn't be until I got home from work some six hours later, that the reality of the entire situation hit me. It had a devastating effect on my self-esteem and confidence. *Had he already blabbed to everyone about my secret and now everyone was going to be looking at me differently? With pity – Ah, I hate pity. Empathy yes, but someone pitying me, no way. Were they going to write me out of the storyline?* **OMG – what if the press finds out!**

I thought about going to Wes, but that would create more drama. I thought even though the director had discovered my secret, which tapped into my deepest fears because he had a reputation for being a tyrant, I also knew he had three young girls at home. I felt that on some level he would connect with my embarrassment, find compassion, and keep my secret. Or at least that's what I had prayed for.

Upon seeing him the next day, he acted like nothing ever happened; and I wasn't surprised. As prefaced earlier, this is a common way of life in Hollywood. I decided it was best not to mention anything or even try to make light of it. He decided to play stupid and I played right along, which was fine with me.

My mother would once again offer me her wonderful perspective in times like this, quickly reminding me of all the positive things I had to be grateful for; okay, so no hair. But, as she would proudly repeat, I was much *more* than hair. It was then that I had one of my more powerful epiphanies. I realized that, even with knowing my secret, that director couldn't take anything away from me because he could never take my essence, my spirit, or sense of self and who I was; with or without a wig. It was a moment in time that could've just as easily been forgotten. My mother would add her solution, "Amy, send it back from whence it came."

And so I did... But ohh, it wasn't easy. It took many, many conversations with myself aloud. Questioning, arguing with mirror... Before I would – or could – find some peace in that moment.

I hoped that whatever was attached to that experience would dissolve over time.

However, I also knew he had his job to protect and it would be stupid to jeopardize that. As always, she had great insight when it came to things that would arise from this issue with me; and she was right. She always made whatever difficulties I was having, *okay.*

The last day on this show was a like a reprieve; a breath of fresh air. I could start new, somewhere else.

On with the adventure.

AFFIRMATION

*The more I love and appreciate myself,
the more beautiful I am becoming.*

Betrayal

*"God, grant me the serenity
to accept the things I cannot change,
the courage to change the things I can,
and the wisdom to know the difference."*

Reinhold Niebuhr

Let me begin with the fact that this was not an easy chapter for me to write. I love my father and over the years we have shared some very special moments. In many ways he has been a good father. Unfortunately there have also been years filled with severe dysfunction, betrayal, pain and abuse.

It was a difficult decision to write deep negativity about my personal relationship with my father. Hurting anyone, including him, is not my goal. At the same time, the nature and timing of this abuse makes it imperative that I speak my truth. Especially if these revelations are to realize their intention, which is to help women connect with their personal strength, overcome their fears and establish true balance and power in their own lives.

The abuse I suffered caused me years of agonizing stress, something no child should ever be subjected to. Most days and nights from 7-16 years old, I was racked with anxiety wondering if my father would come into my bedroom or when the next escapade would occur. There is a direct link between stress, physical, psychological and emotional, to Alopecia. I suffered all, severely for nine years. My Alopecia erupted in the middle of this time frame. It's impossible to separate the two.

For those people who may have judgment or anger about my revealing this part of my life and relationship, I hope they at least understand why I find it necessary to 'come clean.' If there is one person sitting in their room, unable to move forward and feeling worthless, completely unattractive, unworthy and uncomfortable in their own skin as I was; and through this book, they are able to find some traction, experience some peace, hope and inner power again – then I will have contributed what I intended and this disclosure will be the benefit I pray it is.

My father's mother, Grandma Sarah, was a midwife who sold pantyhose and delivered homemade chicken soup to the homeless. Ironically, after her husband died, she could not afford to keep her children. At 5 years old my father and his siblings, two sisters and one brother, were placed in an orphanage. My grandmother's weekly visits were heartbreaking for all of them. They all suffered greatly on many levels.

There are many times my father has shared with me the sexual abuse he incurred by his older brother. I assume at that time it was unspeakable to discuss such things so he kept his silence for many years. It is said that oftentimes, sexual abuse is a multi-generational family issue.

There was one man she considered marrying but he would take only two of her four children, so she never remarried. My Aunt Georgia was the first to get out, singing on the road at age 14. From there, she ultimately experienced many years of great stardom as the #1 singer in the 1950's known as, "Her Nibs Georgia Gibbs." However, she never forgot her suffering and always took care of her mother and a great love of my life, Grandma Sarah. Among many gifts, Georgia made sure to buy her a fur coat before she even purchased one for herself. All opinions about fur aside, at that time, this was a great gesture of love and respect.

I had a deep connection to Grandma Sarah and admired her strength. I was only six years old when she passed away, was heartbroken and often wondered what it would have been like to grow up around such a dedicated, kind, selfless person. As opposed to my Father, who possessed a split personality and vacillated constantly and unpredictably between being an antisocial, judgmental, raging maniac – to a loving, supportive dad who was generous, caring and a great provider. He was also a predator, obsessed with sex, something that got worse as he aged.

Sunday's were spent with many guests, hanging around our Roman-shaped pool, surrounded by the matching shaped bed of roses and a brick wall with a two-room cabana. Everyone would eat Filet Mignon, while admiring my Father's splendid landscaping talents. People were amazed that he was able to turn the original swamp grounds that existed when he first purchased the home, into this magnificently beautiful environment. Most people accepted my father's antisocial behavior and uncontrolled temper as a personality defect and turned their attention to my mom and the other guests.

Prior to marrying my Mom, my father donated his sperm three times to a doctor friend with a patient whose husband was infertile. He became the biological father of three blonde, tow-head boys and apparently always wanted a boy. So I became the boy he and my mother never had. Hence, 'Sports' was my middle name. Golf was his favorite sport and shortly became mine as I was born with a natural talent and a beautiful swing.

Ever since I can remember, I held a club. My father had putting greens around the living room and we would challenge each other to "sink a smooth one." His dream was for me to be the next Cathy Fisher, the lead female golfer in the world at that time. One of the best gifts I ever received was the putter and wood he gave me for my 7th birthday, along with private lessons with a well-known PGA golf Pro named Al who worked at the local golf range a mile from my home. Golf bonded my father and I in a healthy way.

Sex, Wigs and Whispers

Al was 52, in pretty good shape, although at times you could see a little beer belly and then within weeks it would be gone. He was a very structured individual and serious when it came to teaching. He referred to me as the next 'U.S. golf sensation' and how "I could take this kid to the top."

The next several years were spent training to join the Women's PGA. My dad, Al and I, assumed I'd end up in Florida as a world-class golf pro. Al was gregarious, funny, sensitive and caring. I felt like I could share anything with him and never be judged (well, almost anything...). No matter how many bad golf shots I did on an off day, he would help me until I got it right. When I had one of those days, he would be sure to never end our session on a negative. He made me shoot over and over; until I conquered the problem and succeeded at getting even one shot right before ending our lesson. He knew if we didn't, I would obsess on the negative until our next time together. Al truly understood me, unconditionally. He never judged me.

Alternately, while I was the apple of my father's eye, nothing I did was ever good enough for him... ever. He reminded me weekly, that I was always a little too fat or never smart enough. I mirrored my mother's body, especially her tushie and thighs. He insisted I swim 25-50 laps a day to stay in shape and would praise me when I finished. He was irritated and upset when I did not do my daily exercise. As I look back, a little too much so. My sister's physique took after my father's with a more athletic build. I have always wished I could have been born with her long beautiful 'shiksa' legs. Swimming to this day has been part of her daily regimen. Dad was always very health conscious. What kept him in good shape was working hard in the garden and maintaining the grounds and the immense amount of walking he did every day to the train station and back and throughout

Manhattan, buying merchandise for the women's apparel stores he and my mother owned.

Being born with a slight touch of dyslexia made school, especially reading, always a challenge for me; while golf was a place I could soar. I loved all sports. I would ride my bike to the golf range three or four times each week. It was one mile from my house and we would practice two hours, usually leaving me quite sore the next day. It was a place that made me feel special and not less than and I loved the mental and physical challenge. Unlike school, golf came extremely easy to me and I received support and tremendous accolades. Golf was not the go-to sport for most kids. Because there only existed a fruit stand, country club and golf range, many great golfers like Ben Crenshaw were born out in lil' ole' Westchester. I would watch other kids ride their bikes past the golf range, and have a momentary pang, wishing I were doing what they were. In the end, what I kept thinking I wanted was to be normal, like every other kid and family. But I wasn't and we weren't.

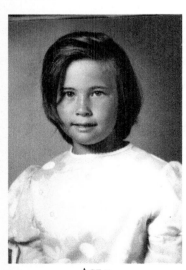

AGE 7

I was 7 years old when there was the first incident. He came into the bathroom after my bath. He didn't behave like a father. I was paralyzed with shock and had no idea how to react, respond or what to feel. One part of me was totally thrown and knew this was wrong; part of me was afraid; while another part of me wanted to please him. I could feel my body begin to react to these very strange and wild sensations. I was shaking with my

Sex, Wigs and Whispers

mind going 100 MPH wondering what would happen next, what could I do... Then, he turned and said, "You are so beautiful, so very special."

I just stared at him.

"Now you know this is our little secret, OK?"

I stuttered, confused, "Uh... yep."

He left. I stayed in the bathroom, staring at the mirror, consumed with a tumultuous confusion, nowhere to turn and no way to comprehend what had just happened to me.

That night, I couldn't sleep, while what had happened churned in my heart and soul most of the night. *Do I tell someone? He said it was "our secret." What did he mean? Is he going to approach me again?* **What do I do now?** Finally, exhausted, I fell asleep.

When I woke up in the morning I was plainly in full denial as I had mercifully blocked thinking about it from my mind. He came downstairs, kissed me hello as usual and we all ate breakfast. But then, something telling happened; I spilled the Orange Juice!

"OH NOOOO" my father bellowed.

I looked at him, jumped up, quickly, apologized to everyone and helped clean it up. After that morning, I spilled my OJ almost every day, for years.

I also began to wet my bed. Looking back years later, I realized these were clear signs that something deep within me was twisting in an attempt to send a 'message in a bottle.' One would think someone would have at least wondered. But

Betrayal

everyone was so busy working all the time, that no one paid attention to these as signs of any problem or of anything deeper going on. Certainly no one in my family bothered to investigate it. I believe these 'repeated incidents' were just considered growing pains in their eyes.

His rages were so intense and frightening; I would hyperventilate in fear and anguish. We would be sitting around the dinner table and out of nowhere he would scream, "Slow down, you're eating too fast! Like a pig. Where were you brought up, in a barn?!"

I would just freeze until his storm blew over.

At night he would come into my room to make sure I had turned my head over to brush my hair because as he would say, "This way the blood will reach your follicle and you will always have a healthy head of hair. Trust me." *Little did he or any of us know.*

About six months later, my father and I were watching the Mets playoffs in our living room. We were alone. My dad had a beer and asked me if I wanted to try it – just a sip. I loved it. As usual, we had a great time rooting for our favorite players. It was our special time. Then, in the middle of the 7th inning, it happened again, only with more urgency. This time it was more physical. I was scared at first, but again was frozen with confusion and didn't know what to do, so I went along with it.

At the end, once again, he turned to me and said, "Thank you baby."

It was incomprehensibly strange. I was numb and afraid to say anything. I again felt like I was in shock. I was only 7 ½ years old. I had no possible way to process any of what had happened. Nothing made any sense to me. I got up and went to the bathroom. And again, I didn't know what to do, what I should do or what

Sex, Wigs and Whispers

would happen next. So I walked back to the living room, sat down on the sofa, leaving some distance between us. He said,

"Oh, come here Ame. It's ok." So I did. I was totally disoriented.

It was surreal – although he didn't miss a beat. We went right back to watching the game as if nothing had happened. Actually, I remember thinking that there seemed to be less stress – an ease about him that had not been present earlier. And it seemed in an odd way that we had a better connection. So I went right along.

So young.

But something did happen. Over and over again and it went on for years. Each time he would stress that this was our secret and no one could ever know. Though I had no idea at the time, I was caught in the dark web of the denial of sexual abuse.

Some of the thoughts I *could* entertain were that I wondered if other kid's dads did the same thing with them, but obviously I dare never ask. What if they didn't? Then what would happen? They would probably tell their parents and then everyone would know! All the kids would think I was weird or something.

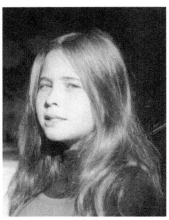

AGE 12 – YOU CAN SEE MY PAIN HERE

And my father would be really angry with me. So, I stayed in my confused and ashamed silence. For years.

Usually it happened at night while my mother was out playing bridge and the maid and my sister were gone. The more I went along with him, the better our relationship *seemed* to be. There was never any kissing, nor was there any other intimacy.

I refused and was deathly afraid to tell anyone anything, including my mother. I was 13 ½ years old and on my first soap opera, *Love of Life,* when I first spoke about it to anyone. I became close friends with the production assistant and one evening during a heart-to-heart talk at her house, I told her the truth about my father. After I had finished crying, thinking I would get a supportive hug and some desperately needed advice, I instead received the opposite. She freaked out and stuttered that she could not discuss any of this with me anymore and ended the discussion. I was heartbroken and shattered, and left abruptly.

She kept her distance from me the entire remaining three years I was on the show. As this incident verified my fears of being ostracized and seen as 'unclean' if I talked about my abuse with anyone, it would be many years before I would tell another soul. Girlfriends that know me now and knew me then, said that they thought something was odd about me; but never knew what to say or do.

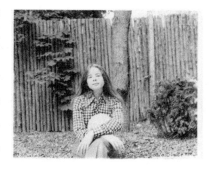

Finally… I figured a way out. At 16½ years old, I cut my finger, rubbed the blood on my underwear and told the maid I got my menstrual period. This gave me the nerve to say to my father, "Well, now that I'm a woman you can't do this to me anymore. I'm not a child anymore."

Miraculously and gratefully, he stopped. The truth is, I did not actually begin my menstrual cycle until I was almost 18 years old, delayed from all of the steroid shots I had been given for my hair loss since I was 13 ½ years old. But I'd found a way out.

Ultimately when I did tell my Mother, she directly filed for divorce.

As the years went on, my 'relationship' with my father grew more intense, as did his severe judgment of me. My ass wasn't small enough, my legs weren't thin enough, or I wasn't smart enough... that one was his favorite.

"You are so stupid! You're such an idiot! You don't even read the newspaper!"

It would take to the age of 35 before I had the nerve to draw a boundary for myself, finally admonishing, "If you tell me how stupid I am one more time I will never speak to you again."

Looking back now, I see how debilitated I'd become emotionally and psychologically. All of what I'd been through with him had taken its toll.

Yet, as he continued this verbal assault on me, I *did* stop speaking to him (this would be merely the first time I cut off communication as a self-defense) and it would be 2 ½ years before I would allow him to be in my life again.

In between his abusing me, my life around him was like sitting on a time bomb and never knowing when it was going to blow. When he wasn't biting my head off, ridiculing me or sexually molesting me, he was acting with full-on charm, and genuine fatherly love, which further confused me, by constantly telling me how beautiful I was and how special my features were or boasting about my acting talents; or over flattering me on my amazing sales expertise in the stores they owned. I enjoyed how close this made us feel – in those moments – and how much he supported me. I know I was starved for approval. At the same time there was a kind of closeness, even though I knew it was strange and conditional. The temporary kindnesses settled my heart – and my nerves; and gave a young girl moments with a Father who cared about her – in a normal way.

Much later in life, as I began the process of healing, I realized my father was in love with me. He treated me like a lover and sadly, hated me like a lover; especially when I 'left' him. He would become jealous of other men looking at me or me looking at them. I remember one day when I went to visit him in San Diego, I was headed to the bathroom, when I was stunned by his contorted reflection in the mirror; he was staring at what he thought was my oversized ass, in utter disgust. I felt so ugly, like I wanted to just crawl into a shell. I immediately made the excuse that I was tired and it was best I left before it got dark. God forbid I would be stuck there! Except that it was only 2 pm. I left and remember driving in silence on the 2 ½ hour stretch back to Los Angeles; feeling like a dark cloud had permeated my soul. The reflection of his face in that mirror exuding such disapproving judgment stayed with me vividly, for weeks; and in truth, far longer.

Over the years many people have asked me, "Why didn't you stop him?"

Why? Because a part of me, I now have come to realize, had become entangled and trapped in a sea of confusion, secrecy and denial. I believed I was supposed to do this because somehow if I didn't obey and comply, then I would lose his love and our relationship – I would lose a Father.

And he would be right there implying that it would be a problem if I didn't do his bidding. I was a very young girl, I believed he was my father and 'father knows best.' At the same time a part of me knew it was very wrong, yet it also gave me some kind of

Sex, Wigs and Whispers

unspoken power that I wasn't willing to give up; maybe some feeling of control in an out of control circumstance. Perhaps this is why I successfully used my sexuality for many years in order to get what I wanted from men. I became aware of this at an early age and had become good at it. Many women may do this, but I had a focal point, a real driver – and I knew it worked.

Although confident and sexually manipulating men on the outside, privately I would gag, often run and throw up when any man actually placed his mouth on my breasts. My real ability to be genuinely intimate and sexual was, at a minimum, scarred.

Throughout my life, even though there have been many times I didn't like my father, and in fact hated him, I've never stopped loving him.

I understand some may not be able to comprehend this and react with: "How can you even speak to someone who crossed such boundaries and did such unspeakable acts to you, never the less still love about him?"

I understand their feelings. However on a spiritual level he, like all of us, is here on the human level working through his own issues. To me, he is a troubled soul and also someone I've learned life lessons from – one way, and another.

It is said, "That which does not kill you, makes you stronger." I am grateful for the strength and courage I've developed in my life; overcoming this experience has contributed to this and to who I am today as a strong and compassionate woman.

I am grateful for and indebted to the many good therapists I have had over the years that have helped me gain clarity and move beyond this abuse. Through much personal growth work

I have been able to move through the scars and enjoy a healthy sex life and a deep level of intimacy.

For a long time, I tried to rationalize his behavior but had never really forgiven him. I thought, no matter what, he was my Father, so I was always supposed to have a relationship with him. Again, I believe that was the guilt talking... Now, I have come to understand that people do the best they can with the tools given them – which is also what makes this type of person so dangerous to be around.

I have learned to take care of me and do what is best for me. I make choices for my own life, in all areas of my life, including this revealing, which supports a higher good in me. It's been a long time since I have had any type of a relationship with my father. As I was going through the process of ending whatever we had, I learned even more about his sexual perversions and am grateful always, that I came through this as well as I have.

My prayer is that any other women who've suffered through this type of experience and are reading this story, may benefit in some way from the disclosure by at least knowing that healing is possible.

STATISTICS AND RESOURCES:

- Children – 15% of sexual assault and rape victims are under age 12.

- 29% are age 12-17.

- 44% are under age 18.

- 80% are under age 30.

- 12-34 years old are the highest risk years.

- Girls ages 16-19 are four times more likely than the general population to be victims of rape, attempted rape, or sexual assault. 7% of girls in grades 5-8 and 12% of girls in grades 9-12, said they had been sexually abused.

- 3% of boys grades 5-8 and 5% of boys in grades 9-12 said they had been sexually abused.

- In 1995, local child protection service agencies identified 126,000 children who were victims of either substantiated or indicated sexual abuse.

- Of these, 75% were girls.

- Nearly 30% of child victims were between the age of 4 and 7. 93% of juvenile sexual assault victims know their attacker.[1]

- 34.2% of attackers were family members.

- 58.7% were acquaintances. Only 7% of the perpetrators were strangers to the victim.

- A study reported in the New York Times suggests that one in five adolescent girls become the victims of physical or sexual violence, or both, in a dating relationship. (New York Times 8/01/01)

- 93% of juvenile sexual assault victims know their attacker. 34.2% of attackers were family members and 58.7 were acquaintances. (U.S. Bureau of Justice Statistics. Sexual Assault of Young Children as Reported to Law Enforcement 2000.

. . . .

1   http://www.feminist.com/antiviolence/facts.htm

NSVRC: National Sexual Violence Resource Center

http://www.nsvrc.org/projects/child-sexual-assault-prevention/
preventing-child-sexual-abuse-resources

RAINN: Rape Abuse & Incest National Network

http://centers.rainn.org

https://www.rainn.org/get-help/local-counseling-centers/state-
sexual-assault-resources

National Suicide - 1-800 Suicide (784 2433)

Nationwide Suicide Hotline - 1-800- 448-3000

The Refuge

http://www.therefuge-ahealingplace.com/ptsd-treatment/child-
sexual-abuse

Recovery.org

http://www.recovery.org/topics/addiction-and-domestic-violence-
or-sexual-abuse/

http://www.recovery.org/topics/choosing-the-best-inpatient-
sexual-abuse-and-addiction-recovery-center/

KCSARC.ORG: King County Sexual Assault Resource Center

http://www.kcsarc.org/gethelp

The National Center For Victims of Crime

https://www.victimsofcrime.org/help-for-crime-victims/get-help-
bulletins-for-crime-victims/bulletins-for-teens/sexual-assault

National_Child_Sexual_Abuse_Helpline.htm

From anywhere in the U.S. call the National Sexual Assault Hotline at 1-800-656-HOPE(4673) or call 202-544-3064 to reach the RAINN business office.

Alabama Coalition Against Rape

Montgomery, AL: 334-264-0123

Alaska Network on Domestic Violence & Sexual Assault (ANDVSA)

Juneau, AK: 907-586-3650

Arizona Sexual Assault Network (AzSAN)

Phoenix, AZ: 602-258-1195

Arkansas Coalition Against Sexual Assault

Fayetteville, AR: 479-527-0900

CALCASA Rape Prevention Resource Center

Sacramento, CA: 916-446-2520

Colorado Coalition Against Sexual Assault

Denver, CO: 303-861-7033

Connecticut Sexual Assault Crisis Services (CONNSACS)

East Hartford, CT: 860-282-9881

Contact Lifeline

Wilmington, DE: 302-761-9800

DC Rape Crisis Center

Washington, DC: 202-232-0789

Florida Council Against Sexual Violence

Tallahassee, FL: 850-297-2000

Georgia Network to End Sexual Assault (GNESA)

Atlanta, GA: 404-815-5261

Guam Healing Arts Crisis Center
Tamuning, GU: 671-647-5351

Hawaii State Coalition for the Prevention of Sexual Assault
Honolulu, HI: 808-733-9038

Idaho Coalition Against Sexual & Domestic Violence (ICASDV)
Boise, ID: 208-384-0419

Illinois Coalition Against Sexual Assault (ICASA)
Springfield, IL: 217-753-4117

Indiana Coalition Against Sexual Assault
Indianapolis, IN: 317-423-0233

Iowa Coalition Against Sexual Assault (ICASA)
Des Moines, IA: 515-244-7424

Kansas Coalition Against Sexual & Domestic Violence
Topeka, KS: 785-232-9784

Kentucky Association of Sexual Assault Programs
Frankfort, KY: 502-226-2704

Louisiana Foundation Against Sexual Assault (LAFASA)
Hammond, LA: 985-345-5995

Maine Coalition Against Sexual Assault
Augusta, ME: 207-626-0034

Maryland Coalition Against Sexual Assault
Silver Spring, MD: 301-328-7023

Jane Doe Inc. / MCASADV
Boston, MA: 617-248-0922

Men Can Stop Rape

Washington, DC: 202-265-6530

Michigan Coalition Against Domestic & Sexual Violence

Okemos, MI: 517-347-7000

Minnesota Coalition Against Sexual Assault

St. Paul, MN: 651-209-9993

Mississippi Coalition Against Sexual Assault

Jackson, MS: 601-948-0555

Missouri Coalition Against Domestic and Sexual Violence

Jefferson City, MO: 573-634-4161

Montana Coalition Against Domestic Violence and Sexual Assault

Helena, MT: 406-443-7794

Nebraska Domestic Violence/Sexual Assault Coalition

Lincoln, NE: 402-476-6256

Nevada Coalition Against Sexual Violence

Las Vegas, NV: 775-355-2220

New Hampshire Coalition Against Domestic & Sexual Violence

Concord, NH: 603-224-8893

New Jersey Coalition Against Sexual Assault

Trenton, NJ: 609-631-4450

New Mexico Coalition of Sexual Assault Programs

Albuquerque, NM: 505-883-8020

New York State Coalition Against Sexual Assault

Albany, NY: 518-482-4222

New York City Alliance Against Sexual Assault
New York, NY: 212-229-0345

North Carolina Coalition Against Sexual Assault
Raleigh, NC: 888-737-CASA (2272)

North Dakota Council on Abused Women's Services/ CASAND
Bismarck, ND: 701-255-6240

Ohio Alliance to End Sexual Violence
Cleveland, OH: 888-886-8388

Oklahoma Coalition Against Domestic Violence and Sexual Assault
Oklahoma City, OK: 405-524-0700

Oregon Coalition Against Domestic and Sexual Violence
Portland, OR: 503-230-1951

Pennsylvania Coalition Against Rape (PCAR)
Enola, PA: 717-728-9740

Day One
100 Medway Street
Providence, RI 02906
401-421-4100
401-454-5565 (fax)
E-mail: info@DayOneRI.org

South Carolina Coalition Against Domestic Violence & Sexual Assault
Columbia, SC: 803-256-2900

South Dakota Coalition Against Domestic Violence & Sexual Assault

Pierre, SD: 605-945-0869

Tennessee Coalition Against Domestic and Sexual Violence

Nashville, TN: 615-386-9406

Texas Association Against Sexual Assault

Austin, TX: 512-474-7190

Utah Coalition Against Sexual Assault

Salt Lake City, UT: 801-322-1500

Vermont Network Against Domestic Violence and Sexual Assault

Montpelier, VT: 802-223-1302

Virginia Sexual and Domestic Violence Action Alliance

Charlottesville, VA: 434-979-9002

Richmond, VA: 804-377-0335 (v/tty)

Washington Coalition of Sexual Assault Programs

Olympia, WA: 360-754-7583

West Virginia Foundation for Rape Information and Services

Fairmont, WV: 304-366-9500

Wisconsin Coalition Against Sexual Assault

Madison, WI: 608-257-1516

Wyoming Coalition Against Violence & Sexual Assault

Laramie, WY: 307-755-5481

PART

2

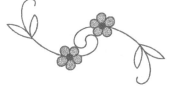

Emotional

Realities

Pitfalls

OUR LIVES ARE THE STORIES WE TELL OURSELVES

Two things define you:
Your patience when you have nothing.
Your attitude when you have everything.

Anonymous

There are common pitfalls that most women fall into...

Losing your hair can be devastating and extremely traumatic. At the same time, feeling this way about the experience begins with the "story" we tell ourselves about what's happening to us and then, this story controls our emotions.

Our minds can run wild when we are vulnerable and this can then lead to our feeling desperate. It's difficult to step outside of a deep emotional experience; it takes help and practice to gain a clearer perspective. Regrettably, the greater the emotional reaction, the greater the distress.

"I'm losing my hair, I'll end up ugly, no one will love me; I'm going to lose my job, everyone will think I'm dying and I'll be left all alone," makes a woman attached to the 'story' she has sold herself. At times like this, it's important to get a reality check from someone you trust; one who knows you well and can help you stay grounded.

A different example would be to cultivate the ability to be an Observer; one who is able to put some space between themselves and the emotional charge of the situation. This perspective enables a Response instead of a Reaction.

"I understand that I have a condition; it may or may not be permanent. But all I can do is stay calm, be pro-active, and do whatever I can to figure to this out. And if I have to get a wig-so be it. I'm not attaching myself to every hair strand that's falling out of my head. I have to still live my life."

This responsive person is more adept naturally at moving through the process of living with hair loss; which is why for some, losing their hair – it's simply just that; a process by which their hair is falling out. They see clumps in the shower, on their pillow, even

Sex, Wigs and Whispers

falling into their soup. But this responsive group of women walks through the experience without the paralyzing depression that hits those of us that are more reactive. They are more resourceful and move on to the next thing they have to deal with and do in their life, period. They don't allow the level of negative emotions others attach to the process, because their 'story' is simply about an 'event.' They take on the role of Observer. I used to think, *"How can someone do that? I'm a mess."*

For yet other women, their flowing mane represents their identity, their sexuality, their sensuality, their ultimate beauty and is their crowning glory. They spend a fortune on shampoos, special treatments, the best brushes and would never ever share their sacred hair secrets. This is the group I belonged to for years, until I got a handle on *my* story and how attached I was to my hair.

We must be clear; my point is not that one story is better than the other. What matters most, is your emotional *responsiveness* instead of *reactiveness* to whatever stories you create for your life. It always comes down to our perception of the stories we tell ourselves. I learned that when I changed my perception, I changed my reality. And if you don't already do this, I believe you will shortly.

It took a while for me to understand this and to get clarity on the role my hair has played in my life. After much inner work, I've come to realize that for me, wigs are accessories, just like the high heels and the makeup I choose to put on to add to my essence.

Even today with as much as I have learned on this journey, I am still stunned when a client walks in the door with the strength and fortitude to walk around in public completely bald, wearing no wig or scarf. I give her so much credit.

Although I believe that "we are more than just hair," personally, I feel better, more beautiful, sexier and more powerful with my hair on. It is for this reason that I have never gone out in the mainstream or taken off my wig in public or in the mainstream media until recently on my live web television show Don't Wig Out! (Vimeo.com/DontWigOut). It took several months before I had the nerve to do it.

Due to the content of this particular show, I felt it was important to share this part of myself with my audience. It was a very liberating experience. However when we were off air and getting ready to go, I was sure to put my beautiful hair back on. The moment I did, it felt like I was home again. Maybe one day this will change for me, but for the moment I'm honoring my process.

There are many shows that have asked me to "GO BALD" simply to add sensationalism to their raise show ratings during "Sweeps" week,[1] with complete disregard for my feelings and that of so many other women who are living with hair loss. It is because of this that I have refused.

I would only agree to expose myself when the content and point of view of the interview is one of integrity and heart. This allows me the opportunity to speak to women directly; where the interviewer understands our plight and is authentic in their caring about hair loss and self-image, and the women living with it. Only recently did I finally decide to do this for a special reality segment on Entertainment Tonight with renowned Beverly Hills plastic surgeon Dr. Brent Moelleken, in step to be an example of what's possible for women with no hair. He is a true artist who understands our sensitivity. It was an extraordinary experience.

. . . .

1   Sweeps is a process by which the networks decide which shows to keep on the air based on numbers of viewership.

Sex, Wigs and Whispers

Through the years, there have been many women who have come to me with stage-one or stage-two cancer. I spent time explaining and preparing them emotionally for their hair loss process and trying on wigs. For these women, losing their hair was so devastating they could not see beyond it and as a result, they chose not to purchase a wig. I was never offended, as I have always believed that those whom I am supposed to help find me at the perfect time. However, these same women came back to me a year or so later, in stage-four cancer. They had ignored whatever chemotherapy treatment was prescribed, in large part because they didn't want to lose their hair. At the beginning of this chapter, I said that our stories and our perceptions of them create our lives, sometimes enabling vulnerable situations to become desperate. This is the extreme example of that mind set and condition. All of these women had families and friends that loved and needed them. Their crowning glory, for some, until too late, was more important – than living. No judgments; I completely understand their fear.

As women, losing our hair can be a crushing experience, beyond belief and paralyzing, even when faced with a life threatening illness.

However, there are those times when we must be realistic and tell ourselves an 'alternate story' and do whatever it takes to stay alive and get healthy; not *only* for ourselves, but for those who love us and depend on our survival. So ladies, no matter what we're faced with – *we* control our choices, we must not allow our stories to dictate our choices. *We* can *change* our stories and our perceptions – in a 'heartbeat.' Each one of us is more powerful than we ever dreamed possible. It is for all women that I chose to tell my story.

AFFIRMATION

I am in control of my condition.
My condition doesn't control me.

Sex, Wigs and Whispers

Understanding Men

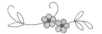

When you find yourself cocooned in isolation and cannot find your way out of the darkness, remember that this is similar to the place where caterpillars go to grow their wings.

Unknown

There are only two types of men when it comes to a woman's hair loss, and there is no in-between:

1) *The Man Who Notices Picky Details;* mostly physical appearances, especially in the woman he's with, he just loves to be right. Often nicknamed 'anal', everything has its place and fits neatly in a compartment. Anything outside of its appropriate box doesn't usually find a place in this man's life, at least not initially. If you find yourself beginning a relationship with this type of man and he is wondering about your hair, he will find all the angles to question you about your 'hair' and won't stop until he forces you to give in; which after reading this book is the last thing you'll do. Whatever you say or do about your hair, will be your choice!

2) *The Man Genuinely Caught Up in You;* he is captivated by your essence, and has more depth. He is so caught up in *you* and *your energy,* that your secret is the last thing he would ever pick up on and the least important thing that he would focus on.

I've experienced both.

These categories are for men you're just meeting. If you are already in a relationship, it is completely different because there is a history; a present and a future that you have created. Bottom line: if you are in an existing relationship and your guy has a problem with your wig, the 'How To's in this book can help you.

But, you may also need a little support from a therapist. Or perhaps you gained enough inner strength and understanding of your own power to simply say, `Hasta Mañana, Baby!'

Sex, Wigs and Whispers

I hope by the time you've finished reading this book, you'll know how to handle these experiences (should they ever arise) while remaining authentic *and* in control of your secret. Hopefully, you won't be consumed with approval of what a man is thinking, or not thinking of you, because you wear hair. Instead, perhaps you'll be at peace with your hair loss and if not, you will have the tools to feel confident enough to act as though you have a natural, full head of hair. This gives you the opportunity to have a genuine experience with this person; one focused on who the two of you really are, and not on your hair (or lack of it) or your fears around that. There's plenty of time to share your emotions about your hair loss later, when both of you are ready, should you get there.

Men do one of nine things when it comes to hair loss. They:

- Get intrigued
- Become scared
- Act loving
- Get angry
- Feel powerless
- Run
- Fix It (or try to)
- Become supportive
- Get strong

But one thing is for sure after reading this book: You will have the opportunity to still be standing strong and proud regardless of his reactions. Even the most supportive man will initially have one of these responses because men are 'solutionists,' which is one of the differences in how men and women listen to and process information. When any man sees or hears about a problem, his initial reaction is to start thinking of a way he can fix the situation. The wise man knows he does this.

Many of my clients are cancer patients and most men find this disease more complicated to deal with than the hair loss that often accompanies chemotherapy or radiation treatment. This is largely because it is completely out of their control and they cannot save their loved one from the pain they must endure to hopefully beat this disease. This is of course, the ultimate desired solution. And men have no control of when or if, this terrifying disease will rear its ugly head again, so many men cannot help but feel like a failure.

Sadly, I have met many disappointing partners, husbands and boyfriends of my female clients going through cancer treatment. When I first began my business fifteen years ago, and a client would come in with her partner who acted selfish, harsh and unsupportive, while she was facing this devastating journey, I would get angry. I soon realized that most of the time, it was just that these men were frightened by their lack of control and the inability to find a solution to a devastating situation. Fear makes all of us act in ways we normally would not. They just didn't know how to handle their loved one being sick, and took it out on their partner.

Often, I'll purposely drop a client's wig on the floor and then ask my client's partner to please pick it up – just so he can feel it. Most men are afraid to feel human hair at first; it's a little strange for them. (In fact, it's a little strange for most people at first; myself included). However, touching the wig immediately brings a person's partner into the experience; and makes it real for him in an organic sort of way. As if he is now part of her beautiful transformation, instead of just commenting on how a wig may look on her. After a moment of hesitation they usually concede and it has always proven to have a positive effect on the overall experience.

I have asked many husbands and boyfriends to leave, telling them it would be best for me to work with their wife/girlfriend alone. Then, inevitably after he leaves, she cries; the fear of losing him due to her hair loss is larger than possibly her own mortality. I'm not a therapist; what I offer is compassion, a common understanding and genuine empathy in helping these women.

You will hear me say many times; all women with hair loss are on a courageous and challenging life journey. We have to dig deeper and look beyond our hair or external attributes to find what makes us special.

Women with cancer are facing their own mortality and often losing body parts in addition to their hair. They are faced with having to make serious choices to go through what is necessary to fight and stay here for their loved ones. These women are my heroes.

All women living with hair loss hold a special place in my heart.

Some men hide, some men run; but many men will stay and support you in finding a beautiful *new you*. They'll take the journey *with* you. And even men, who do not start this way out of fear, can turn around. It is truly fabulous when a man is supportive of his woman in this process and together they can make it a fun experience putting on different looks and colors; inevitably touching on their past experiences together, bringing forth wonderful memories and thus enhancing their connection.

Understanding Men

But alas, there have been and still are, men who shock me with their shallowness; only thinking of their sexual attraction and needs at such a frightening time. The thought of their woman not being "whole" without her hair, missing a breast or having scars, or being unable to live their lives "as usual" turns them off. This is largely a reflection of their own insecurities. To me, these men are small... on every level.

And then there are the many wonderful men who stand by their lover's side, praising their partner for the courage she shows while taking on this frightening journey and to look this massive wild animal in the eye, head on without ever backing down, regardless of the fight and the life change it may take to win. This heightens their attraction and takes their relationship to an even deeper level. These men, I love!

The opportunity for any woman facing this journey of hair loss is the discovery that *who you are* is much greater than your hair or your breast. Your spirit is alive and growing, because of and in spite of, your journey; and for the men in these women's lives, it's wondrous to behold and experience.

The depth of a woman far surpasses that of a man in my book. I may make some enemies in saying this – but women have a larger capacity to feel. Men are not inept and without feeling, they just have a few things to turn-off first before they can get to the place women "live" every day. One thing is for sure: When it comes to men, Confidence is the strongest aphrodisiac.

Sex, Wigs and Whispers

1) *Remember if you're calm – they'll be calm. I am not saying that you should disregard your feelings; but for a short amount of time just put them aside, breathe and tell yourself, "I look great, and I'm fine." Acting 'as if' it's already fine, is the only way to true manifestation of that exact reality.*

2) *It helps to ask questions about his life, and then force yourself to get out of your head and get into his – and most of all really...* <u>*listen.*</u> *(Men love a good listener)*

Obviously creating this level of manifestation to achieve the life you want goes way beyond just this example; it's in everything we do. Or shall I say desire.

AFFIRMATION

I only surround myself with people that remind me of my inner strength and beauty.

They Only Get Smart When We Get Stupid

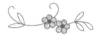

*"I've learned that people will forget what you said,
people will forget what you did,
but people will never forget how you
made them feel."*

Maya Angelou

Help! It's time to go out!

When it comes right down to it, the First Date might be one of the most emotional moments of your entire hair-loss journey. So listen up ladies and Don't Panic! It really will be okay... maybe even great!

They only get smart, when we get stupid.

First, know that most men are basically oblivious when it comes to hair. Yes, with respect to your wig, even Mr. Anal we talked about in the previous chapter really won't notice the details of your hair, until you give him a specific reason to.

We have a tendency to think everyone knows; but most people, especially men, have absolutely no idea you are wearing alternative hair. People/men are generally caught up in themselves and focused on having a good time with you, not staring at your hair. Typically, there is one person that always gives away your secret... *it's you.* Rarely does anyone ever know, unless we actually tell him or her or do something that brings attention to it not being our own hair. It's usually out of our own insecurity and by our own actions, that we give away our secret; and that strange "dance" is activated with the person we are with.

It plays out like this or some variation of this theme:

You go out with someone you're attracted to and you're nervous. You start talking too much–or not at all–you look down while you're talking–or step back a bit while in conversation–or begin playing with your hair–or all of these at the same or different times.

Sex, Wigs and Whispers

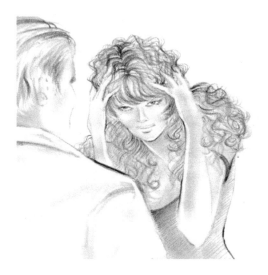

The other person picks up on any of these on an energetic level and gets a bit confused, maybe begins to feel uncomfortable. He unconsciously starts to react to your every move and then you feel him beginning to pull away; all the while your heart is racing so fast it feels like it's jumping out of your chest, which freaks you out more. He reacts to *that* energy and pulls away even further. The vicious cycle continues, until someone bolts as quickly as possible.

Well at least that was my experience for years. I'm not saying that every woman on this hair loss journey has these experiences, but based on the amount of women I have worked with for over 15 years, it is far more common than not.

Even though it's difficult to believe until you actually live with your wig on, you can absolutely do everything without anyone knowing you're wearing a wig… including on a date! It's all up to you.

Believe it or not this little process can work wonders (cultivate this practice, and it gets easier with time). The secret here is about 'stopping' the adrenaline, the emotional spin that we are in or about to enter.

If you're caught off guard and the moment doesn't feel right, take a breath, try to stay calm and tell yourself,

"It's ok." Say your name and repeat, " _____, you're fine. That was just a moment, you're good now." Take a deep breath. Let it out slowly. With a sense of relief, softly say, "I'm good." Now, move on with your day.

If needed, calmly excuse yourself for a moment, go to the nearest bathroom if one is available, and give yourself the time it takes to get centered and be alone with your thoughts. Wait until this feeling of being 'okay' resonates with you and <u>feels</u> real to your core.

If you feel the anxiety begin to creep up, (what I refer to as the "crazies"), just remember to breathe and calmly repeat silently to yourself,

"I'm okay, I just need to take a moment right now. I'll be fine.." And you will be.

Don't worry about what the other person is thinking just stay with concentrating on yourself for the moment. Being still is not a bad thing; it allows us to get centered. Whether you are with people or not, this will always work and give you time to digest the situation and figure out your next move. The only person here is you. The only thoughts that matter are the ones you have about yourself, no one else's judgment. You can do this.

TIP 2: Preparation:

Caution: There is a fine line between being ready and pushing yourself to get there.

There have been times when I have been extremely uncomfortable with someone and had to talk myself into being 'okay' just to get through the moment with that person. Even though my heart was racing, I literally bluffed my way, acting as if I were emotionally 'in control' of the entire situation. Basically, not giving my emotions any life, ultimately forcing myself to move though it. Obviously, I wasn't ready. Yet I still had to move forward with my life for what was needed at the moment.

It was a tough choice; do I stay in my shell or tackle this crazy thing that is literally taking control of my soul and preventing me from having any joy in my life? I just couldn't live any longer in the pain, depression, and frustration. I just had to find a way to get to get back to that feeling of joy and happiness, which at this point was so far removed from my consciousness, it took all my might to bring up any memory of it.

But on the other hand, I knew that because this sense of happiness existed before, I could tap into it if I worked at it.

Sometimes, it took me actually lying to myself; finding every reason to talk myself into literally believing that I was in control of my emotions about my hair loss, to the point of having a sense of calm about it all. I would repeat to myself,

"I got this handled, no biggy."

Oddly enough, this really helped me. Soon, it became innate and I was suddenly comfortable. However, everyone has their own window of time in finding their comfort level.

It's vital that you get a handle on this and figure your comfort level psychologically and emotionally before moving forward. If you choose to bluff, make sure you have your emotions majorly intact before attempting to pull this off. What I mean by that: it's important to understand our limitations and how far we can take them to know the level of inner work that stands in front of us.

How I did this? you ask ...

First, I took a deep breath and then I would slowly release. I would force myself into imagining a beautiful ocean, and the feeling of my feet in the soft warm sand like I felt in Hawaii – thinking anything that would calm me. I keep saying this, but it works. I know it's not always easy, but you can do this "if" you choose to believe you can.

Secondly, I would remind myself of my extraordinary qualities that were hard to find in others. My wit and humor, etc. At times this took a bit of work, as I had to keep telling myself over, and over again,

"I am fine. This hair does not define me. Who I am in my heart, my mind, and my essence is what defines me. No one else owns my wit. No one else sees things exactly as I see them. I am different and I am special. I AM Special."

There were times when I just couldn't get there – just couldn't see past my depression; finding every reason to pick myself apart in the most self-loathing ways imaginable. It was then that I would reach out to a dear friend who would remind me of the qualities I had forgotten about that made me special. Sometimes we need to do this. Decide who that person is for you, that you can totally trust to call upon and who, without question, will *unconditionally remind you of your incredible qualities. Because I believe there is not a woman on this planet who does not possess something special with her own inner spirit that is incomparable to any other.*

As I began to feel more in control and more comfortable in my own skin, I could sense myself feeling my inner power more, so it was easy for me to do step three. That's when I had to just go for it... and get to a place of being okay with this hair loss, this wig process. Again reminding myself, "Amy, it is what it is – stay out of the drama" just keep moving on to the next thing at hand". However, gaining the knowledge I needed about wigs which allowed me to pick the correct style, density, and color for myself was vital in giving me the confidence I needed to move through this dating process successfully. I would frequent many wig shops and ask lots of questions. I wasn't shy as I figured they are in the business of helping people, they should feel comfortable answering my questions. Most stores will make themselves available to your inquiries, especially if they think it will lead to a possible sale.

I would take the wig that interested me out to the natural light instead of depending on the store's fluorescent lighting to make my decision on color. I would make sure to request a "few" minutes with the store stylist so I could get her insight on what cut would look best on me. I was careful not to take advantage of her time and just ask her one or two questions whenever I stopped by, and in a short amount of time she became very generous with her time. Most stylists love transformation and if not with a client, they will gladly help you.

When I did decide to let someone in, it worked out fine. Largely because I took the time to get in control before allowing him access to my secret, and I wasn't looking for anyone's approval of me, which so many of us do who have lost our hair. In my mind he was lucky to have me! Granted, it took some practice before I was able to get to this place! But when I finally got there it was life altering!!

It will be for you too. Just use the tools in this book. You may have heard Eleanor Roosevelt's famous quote;

> **"A woman is like a tea bag. You don't know how strong she is until she is placed in hot water."**

Nothing is closer to the truth.

So, ladies – don't ever forget how wonderful and superior you are. Losing your hair makes you even more special because you're different and deeper than most women. As I've mentioned earlier, those of us who have lost our hair have had to investigate ourselves more than the norm to find out what makes us tick, aside from just our looks.

Try this with me:

Imagine for just a moment that you're looking in the mirror, and just allow yourself to look at your eyes, your lips, your features, one by one. No one else has these but you. Now, *feel* what it's like when you know you look beautiful. When you know you ROCK. That inner *ahhh, yes. I'm looking good!* Now wait – don't allow yourself to go into judgment – stay with that confident feeling right now. Take a deep breath and as you release your breath, feel what it's like to *know* you are on the money, that no one can get close to what you are about.

Now that the feeling is familiar, you can always go to that place when you need to.

It's just taking a moment to get out of the fear, out of your head and back into your heart.

At Agape International Spiritual Center in California, my spiritual home for the last 22 years, we are taught to envision your life the way you want it. Don't try to figure out "how" to get it; just act "as if" it's already happened. Knowing, in the deepest part of your core being, down to the very cellular level, that you already have what you need, that you are already a part of this lifestyle, with whomever you envision being with, and already at whatever job you desire, and in the environment you yearn for.

Then for the secret... now... Know that it's done. Period.

Then let it go and watch what unfolds before you.

When I have truly allowed myself to believe the changes, of what already *has transpired in my life – it has been astonishing. Manifestation is wonderful thing. And anyone can achieve this for anything they desire... if they choose to.*

AFFIRMATION

Losing your hair does not mean
you have lost your essence.
It's who we are embedded deep in our DNA.
Nothing, and no one, can take that away from us.

Date Rape

"When everything seems to be going against you, remember that the airplane takes off against the wind, not with it."

Henry Ford

He was every Jewish mother's dream; a handsome, wealthy, Beverly Hills doctor from a good family and a member of the tribe. I was taken in from our first encounter. Our meeting came at a profoundly conflicted period in my life. New to this journey, I saw myself as a hairless freak, while desperately trying to come off with the outward impression that my looks and my psyche were beautiful. My work demanded this; the entertainment industry centers on physical appearance, self-confidence and is hyper critical in these areas. Looks are money in show business; anyone can *act* confident, but the critical emphasis and importance of physical beauty are why there're so many boob and nose jobs. In reality, I felt like a big nothing… like a deep and aching oblivion in my soul. When I met Sam, I felt a surge of light inside my body; the woman in me was reawakening!

The typical trilogy ensued: our first date was coffee; second, lunch; the big crescendo with our third outing – dinner. With each date our connection grew deeper. At the restaurant during dinner the wine, the food and the romance, fed my 'All-Us-Girls Belief' that the man sitting across from me had it all and I was his special someone. For that evening I was whole, beautiful and worthwhile. Sam was caring, gentle and most importantly, genuinely interested in me. (*I was already picking out my wedding gown!*) Touched, I cautiously shared my deep dark secret – tentatively and directly telling him that, "I had no hair and I was wearing a wig."

Much to my relief Sam didn't flinch and showed no signs of being turned off or repulsed. He was accepting and listened thoughtfully. He was still interested in me. *I was on top of the world.*

Sex, Wigs and Whispers

Naturally, when he suggested we go to his house for a nightcap, I happily accepted. I was surprised at how modest his home was. It lacked the trappings I would have expected from a 'Jewish doctor.' I quickly chalked it up to his having other, more important priorities and in fact, actually thought more highly of him for it. After lighting a fire, he poured me a glass of fine red wine; we settled *into* his sofa and gently fell into a deep embrace. Then he began to sensually remove one bit of clothing after another. The chemistry at this point was very intense and I realized that this adventure was going faster and further than I wanted or was ready for.

Then suddenly, my heart began to pound even more as he reached behind my neck! I slowly moved his hand onto my cheek, kissing all of his fingers, anxious to distract him from my 'hair.' But he was determined and would not stop his pursuit.

Quickly and without warning, he threw me on the floor, pinned me down and tore off all my remaining clothes and jumped on top of me! Almost naked I screamed,

"NO! STOP!"

He ripped off my panties and rapidly thrust himself inside of me, continuing to hold me down with one hand. The other hand RIPPED MY WIG OFF! As he plowed into me like some farm animal he said, *"You know, those little patches of hair are kind of weird looking, you'd look better if you just shaved them off."*

Shocked and consumed with fear, I tried to push him off of me but he would not budge. Gasping for air I had no choice but to let him finish. Once satisfied, he immediately released my body. I took gulps of air while I tried to cover my head, and my body.

Date Rape

Many women experience this because sadly, violating women like this is an all too common component of our world. Women are forced to have sex, even when they say NO, STOP! And for me, it was that much more traumatizing because in addition to this violation, it was the first time any man had ever seen me without my wig! Bald. As a woman, unless you have been bald, you may not understand the depth of this exposure. It was as if I was a virgin being raped!

I believed for years this was all my fault and Sam was excused from any blame on the matter. My thinking was that I had allowed it to get this far, only to cut it off abruptly, in the midst of passion. It took years of therapy and the rebuilding of my self-confidence for me to see absolutely that it was actually *Sam* that had abused *me* and in the worst possible way. __*NO Means NO. Not Maybe.*__

Being raped and having my wig pulled off at the same time gave me the opportunity to learn just how vulnerable a woman is when she's lost her hair. As women, we enter this man's world with a different level of susceptibility. A woman with no hair in a society that is 'hair first' has yet a *deeper* level of susceptibility. This is not a victim flag for any of us or a license to give up! It's just about accepting what is and learning what it takes to move beyond it to achieve our dreams.

It is up to you to be a victim or accept what is. The choice is always yours.

Never share your secret in an emotional moment. All important decisions require and deserve reflection. I did not give sharing my secret with him the consideration it deserved. See the section on Sharing Your Secret.

AFFIRMATION

NO Means NO. Not Maybe.
I am worthy of having people around me that respect, love, and cherish, who I am in my soul.

PART

3

Sharing Your Secret

Sharing Your Secret...
Is Like Sharing
Your Heart

The difference between school and life?
In school, you're taught a lesson
and then given a test.
In life, you're given a test
that teaches you a lesson.

Tom Bodett

I believe in feeling a person out a bit in order to get an understanding of their level of sensitivity.

You may want to first see how they feel about "hair" and the level of importance that it may play in their life 'prior' (*operative word here*) to having 'the discussion.' This way there are no surprises and you can handle the subject matter; your approach will be much easier and more successful. I would be lying if I said that this hair journey has not been both painful and joyous for me. However, I stand here before you completely naked – and hopefully, by allowing you to see into my heart and feel my passion for this journey you'll get solid solutions and peace of mind. The most important question to ask yourself:

Am I READY? Is this the RIGHT TIME to let this person in and my secret out?

Peter was 6'3", blonde (*not my usual type*), very bright and really funny (*always an instant button for me*). It was our first date and I was filled with anticipation. We met on the checkout line at Whole Foods supermarket *(one of the many great "pick up" places in LA)*. From that fateful moment we spoke every night, 15-45 minutes, each conversation bringing us closer together. When he came to the door I had to take a breath, our chemistry was even more palpable than in our first meeting. After one week, it felt like months had flown by between us. In one of our talks he mentioned a surprise for our first date.

Sunset Boulevard was filled with billboards in the sky. Peter took a hard right into the parking lot of a beige building, with female bodies painted on the outside, and a sign that read 'The Body Shop.' His surprise? ...It was really a strip joint. No, I did not ask him to take me home; I did not leave, nor did I even protest.

I was still filled with the insecurity that plagues most women at the beginning of their hair loss journey.

I thought, *"Don't rock the boat – it's going well..."*

Hopefully after reading this book, you can gain your confidence back sooner than I did.

I couldn't believe that he would think that I would agree to all this. Uh uh! Especially on a first date! In a nanosecond, curiosity, fear, excitement and fury were running through my body simultaneously, while at the same time I was trying to keep my cool. Yet there we were – along with the many naked bodies coming my way as we entered. So I made the best of it, as I always do. I embraced my curiosity about the whole place. Three things immediately went through my mind when we walked into the chaos of parading stripped bodies:

1) These women never eat!

2) These women must live in the gym!

3) With legs like that, none of these women are Jewish!

I have met very few of us who have long lanky legs and those little tushies, born naturally thin. God Bless them. I've always dreamed of having long thin tight legs, you know the type that need no pantyhose! If these girls had been thin, it was usually due to excessive dieting, working out, plastic surgery or Liposuction surgery, but of course they would never admit to that. Especially my comrades in Hollywood; they'll go to their graves claiming it's 'natural' and they were 'born that way'. Even a well-known sex icon, an actress in her seventies who has a wig line, the bombshell from all the movies on the big screen, looks like no one has ever touched her face.

But we girls know better... She has not one line on her face and her boobs stand at attention! (God Bless her). Ladies, let's get real: if you're dealing with women, it's best to be authentic. It's much more endearing. However, I admire and believe that women should do whatever it takes to better themselves. And she was ahead of her time; no celebrity would do a wig line! I thank her as she helped pave the way for all of the gals wearing and designing wigs! The hell with what anyone says or thinks. And yes, I have had liposuction, had my boobs done, and had a recent "tune up." *Oh well, what's a girl to do!*

The hostess appeared with of a couple body parts barely covered, a spitting image of the other girls. My curiosity had not yet caught up with my discomfort, and when she turned to walk us to our table – I froze in my tracks. Directly in front of me swayed a back full of the most gorgeous, luscious mane of hair that travelled all the way down the girl's back...just like mine *used* to be. That's when I began to hyperventilate. This was not the first time a gorgeous head of hair stared at me... but never in a situation where I was this self-conscious.

We are, all of us, more vulnerable hiding the secret that we are bald. Still, I never told Peter that anything was wrong. I kept trying to breathe through each moment, which seemed to be endless. I spoke very few words but continued to smile a lot, acting as if I was listening to his every word when in fact, I hardly heard a thing. Finally, I began to calm down, came back into my own skin and was able to enjoy this new experience. What the hell; at the very least I figured this evening would certainly give me some juicy moments to write about in my journal.

After an hour, his suggestion we go to the comedy store was a much-welcomed reprieve. I thought some good laughter might ease the evening's tension. We arrived early, ordered drinks and soon we felt as bonded as when we met and flirted every night on the phone. I quickly forgot about our first, inappropriate stop. Until for whatever the reason and without notice, he suddenly blurted out, "So tell me something, what was the deal with you and the girl with the hair just now at the other place? What was up with that?"

"What do you mean?" I said almost choking on my water before getting the words out.

"Well, it was strange. I mean, one minute you seemed to become almost, I don't know, *fixated* on it; and the next so sullen and closed off. I just don't understand where all that was coming from."

I was a bit taken aback and my first response out of fear was to deny it and pretend I didn't know what he was referring to. But there it was again – that need to be honest – jumping at the right moment to do what I had planned: share my secret, show him who I really was, and be emotionally forthright with him. He would after all, absolutely adore me even more because of what I was courageously enduring.

I opened up about my Alopecia, the whole story and did not even get emotional. I knew from growing up with seven male first cousins who were like my brothers, that men do not do well with too much emotion being thrown at them. Peter stayed completely quiet and really intrigued. After I was finished, he asked for 'a minute to process this' (A usual reaction for men). Even though I was anxious for his response, I felt such fear that I reluctantly gave him the time he needed and remained silent for what seemed like fifteen minutes, but in reality was barely two. To make light of the moment, while he was deep in thought, I began to look around, then back at him, then waited a minute;

and finally, in an obvious and cute way, I pulled out my wrist to look at my watch, and looked him straight in the eye as if to say, "Well?" (with a smile of course).

He thanked me for my honesty and told me he had never heard of this before. He asked a few questions, and again touched on my weird behavior at the strip club toward the hostess. Wow! He *had* noticed. He cared. He congratulated me on my courage;

Whew, he's ok – he gets it.

I was so relieved. He was sweet and continued to compliment me on my beauty, excusing himself politely to go to the men's room. Of course, a thousand things began to run through my head. Even though I had decided to share my story with Peter before he picked me up that night, I questioned if it was too soon. But then again, we felt so connected...how could I not open up?! I wondered if he was really freaked-out, suspicious that all the compliments were just a cover. I noticed fifteen minutes had gone by. I began to feel weird. At twenty minutes I got extremely nervous. At twenty five minutes, I went to the men's room and asked a guy to look in there for him. The men's bathroom was empty. I stood there, my eyes darting around the restaurant. I went out front to look for him but didn't see him anywhere. Finally, I went to the hostess and asked if she had seen my date. She informed me that, "Oh yes, he left and gave the valet his ticket fifteen minutes ago."

LESSONS:

- Sharing your secret does not bond you to anyone.

- Your hair loss should not be used as a way to connect with a man, ever.

Sex, Wigs and Whispers

- The only thing that bonds two people is experience and that takes time.

- This part of you might feel like if you let someone in it will increase the connection, but if it's too soon and you don't receive the reaction your were hoping for, it might feel like they've stabbed you with a knife.

- Make sure you are emotionally prepared on all levels before you make the conscious choice to tell him.

- You don't have to share everything about yourself at the beginning of getting to know someone, especially something as big as hair loss. You are not being dishonest if you do not share your secret right away. This is your body, your mind, your heart. You take all the time you need.

- Sharing your secret is a *gift* you give someone who is *deserving* of it, not used to manipulate the situation – ever. That just gives up your power.

These were great reasons for why I had planned on sharing my secret with Peter on our first date. After all the time we spent talking, there was a definite bond. The truth is, we were not bonded – but we had great chemistry. Big difference. At the end of the day, all I did was set myself up to be hurt. If I had given us time, I would have discovered that Peter was the kind of person who goes to strip joints on the first date and when faced with something he can't handle or doesn't like – he runs away. Our chemistry would have faded as surely as we would have.

Many women feel they would rather be rejected now, than later. If you get to know someone, you will learn if he deserves knowing this part of you. If you decide he does, because of who he is and who you are together, he will embrace you and your secret.

There are some who feel that by a 'certain amount of dates' with a person they have the right to know and should be told because if you don't, you're pretending to be someone you're not. I completely disagree.

You need to give a person time to fall in love with your soul and your heart, so they can get beyond anything out of the norm, like hair loss, which, without having a real degree of trust with a person could become a huge issue. Everyone sizes each other up in the beginning. It's normal – especially in the infatuation stage. We are all seeking our dream mate.

Just think, if you met someone who had many of the elements you are looking for and on the first meeting he tells you his challenges, what he may feel are his imperfections, even if you don't feel that they are, would you be more or less attracted? Half the fun of dating is the courting, the mystery and getting to know someone.

As you're getting to know someone, notice how they feel about 'hair' and the level of importance it may play in their life. Even for a man that has always placed tremendous importance on hair, being with the right woman usually trumps that. Understanding your man gives you the power to share your secret in a way that creates the space for him to appreciate your hair loss journey and at the same time have his feelings about it. And doing it this way does sincerely bring you closer together. More on 'How To' do this in "Broaching the Subject"...

This hair journey story has been both painful and joyous for me. There were solutions and peace, and growth and love. Keep reading...

Sex, Wigs and Whispers

TIP: BOTTOM LINE – Take Your Time.

Rarely do a few, 30-minute phone calls, determine a connection. Time spent with that person is the only way to really assess their character and soul – and, how well you mesh. It would be a while before I would let someone else in again that quickly. But when I did, Ladies – he was worth it. And the reason it went so smoothly when I did tell this other man about my hair loss, was because I had taken the time to get to know him as a friend, truly seeing how I felt with him, and letting him into my heart. Most of all I felt safe... When you take the time, you'll be more in control of your personal power. You'll know when you're ready. Just take the time to listen to your heart and not your head (your heart intelligence is 'smarter,' as is your gut intelligence). And by all means, try to keep your groin out of the process here – until later!

AFFIRMATION

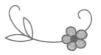

*I am totally in control and have
the ability to follow my instincts.
I listen to my heart with a perfect ear,
and know when it's the right time to let someone in.*

Sharing Your Secret... Is Like Sharing Your Heart

Sex, Wigs and Whispers

Honoring Yourself

*"One important key to success is self-confidence.
An important key to self-confidence is preparation."*

Arthur Ashe

This was something totally unexpected.

Steve and I were on our third date. As always, it promised to be a glorious and fun evening. He did all the right things; showed up with a bouquet of Calla Lilies, my favorite flower; wore a gorgeous, elegant suit that enhanced his handsome looks and chose a romantic restaurant that I had always wanted to dine at. We pulled up to the restaurant and I did the quick glance in the mirror to be sure make-up and hair were in place... I looked hot.

The valet helped me out of his Porsche and Steve came around to escort me up the stairs, arm-in-arm, to the front entrance of the restaurant. Dates were always exciting; and for this one, I starved for two days to fit into my fab leopard outfit! I was famished and ready for what promised to be an amazing meal from one of the best chefs in the country.

As I walked, Steve placed his hand on the small of my back (I've

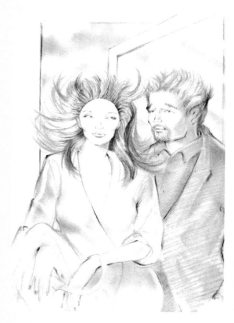

always loved when men do that). But, just as he opened the entrance door for me, a sudden gust of wind came at me so hard that I lost my balance! My hair in the front of my wig lifted up, forcing my wig to fly backward, exposing my wig line!

I froze momentarily, not knowing what to do. This was a first! I immediately looked down and quickly moved the front of my hair back in place.

Sex, Wigs and Whispers

It was obvious by his reaction that Steve had seen my wig, but he was too much of a gentleman to react in any way. By the time we sat down, the change in the vibe between us was palpable. Suddenly, there was a large elephant in the room. Trying to stay cool, I held my fingers tightly under the table and remembered to breathe, like I had been taught to do when nervous and needing to get a grip.

Fortunately, the waitress came over and diverted our attention – a welcomed relief for the moment. After an interminable ten minutes, I decided to broach the subject of his relationship with women, in particular his Mom. I made sure to listen, stay out of my head, be present and just as I suspected – he loved this approach from me. Finally, we were back on track and the energy between us was flowing better. *(More about how you can do this later.)*

In the month we had gotten to know each other, I witnessed Steve's sensitivity to spirituality. I was beginning to feel safe. If this relationship was going to go anywhere, regardless of its label, i.e. friendship or potential husband, I wanted to be honest. I brought up the gust of wind experience and how it almost knocked me over. Then, off handedly I followed it with,

"It knocked me so hard it almost took my new hairdo with it!"

He was shocked by my humor which soon turned into a great laugh. Then, it was time to get real. I broached the subject, told him the truth and made sure to keep it light. He admitted he had never heard of Alopecia before and asked if it was "catchy" or "fatal." I was a bit taken aback for a moment, since this was the first time anyone asked me this question before. It took all my might to sport a calm smile, while I replied,

"No, you won't die if you kiss me!"

Honoring Yourself

He then moved closer, leaned in, held me and gave me the warmest, most loving kiss. Then he said, "It's cool. I bet you look amazing without your hair. I kinda' want to know more – if you're open to talking about it."

So as much as I wanted to relish in the moment of acceptance with Steve, I realized I wasn't equipped to share more with him. I just wasn't emotionally ready. Remember, your guy deserves to know more, but always on *your* terms, when *you're* ready. I decided to honor myself and promised,

"We will; later, just not tonight. Tonight, I was looking forward to hearing some comedy. So let's go laugh."

When the evening ended, we were both happy and light. Over the ensuing weeks however, when I felt a bit safer, I would share more about the condition and the challenges I had endured with it since my youth as a teenager. Within this time, it became clear we would not be together for the long term. We eventually parted ways as friends.

What was most important to me about this experience with Steve was a confirmation that I was finally getting a handle on this issue. And to trust that it's absolutely fine to do things *in my own time and on my terms.* This kept me in my power – not disempowered by someone else's need or timetable. This was a life-changer for me and it can be for you, too.

There are many situations where the wind can catch your hair. Opening a restaurant door, or walking into a building through a moving door are just a few, like it did with Steve. Most importantly, is for you to remain calm and to stay centered. Immediately treat your piece like it's your real hair and no one will ever catch on.

Sex, Wigs and Whispers

If you want to run your hands through your hair — then do it! *Just a bit more gently.*

Over time my piece has become part of me and with a little practice all these techniques worked better and better as I got more comfortable with my hair, myself and the process.

TIP:

A) When walking into the restaurant against a gust of wind lower your head just slightly and tuck your chin down a bit, ever so slightly, the wind will push the top of your hair downward instead of blowing directly into your face and lifting the bangs backwards, thus exposing the frontal line of your wig.

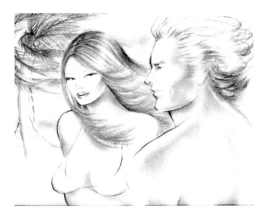

You can use this tip for walking on the beach or wherever you may find yourself in a gust of unexpected wind.

Investing in a good hair system can make all the difference in creating a strong level of comfort. I do love lace front pieces and they work beautifully for those who wear the front of their hair off their face, going backwards. If you're someone who wears your bangs going forward, there is little need for a lace front. However, you can camouflage the front edge of wig by styling baby hair into the wig. (refer to Styling section).

Keep in mind that if you plan on wearing a lace front piece every day, the lace has a tendency to tear and get worn out more quickly than a regular base cap. With constant wear, it may need to be replaced approximately every 4-5 months, which can be costly. Approximate cost for repair can range from $250-$500 dollars.

AFFIRMATION

I own my condition; my condition does not own me.
As I challenge my fears, I am strengthened & empowered.

Sex, Wigs and Whispers

Reality Check

"There is nothing enlightening about shrinking so that other people will not feel insecure around you."

Marianne Williamson,
A Return to Love

Here it is: Female hair loss can be an issue for some men. However, their issues Do Not need to become *your* problem.

Of all the experiences I have been through with men and potential partners, this particular one was life changing for me. It showed me I could stand strong, exactly as I am. It showed me absolutely, that I know my self-worth.

Alan and I had known each other for years in and around Los Angeles. He was wealthy, successful and handsome. He was also known for dating women with beautiful hair.

"No short crop cuts for this guy." His parties were famous, as were his social skills. Charm and panache was this guy's middle name. Many ladies dreamed of being with Alan. I was a successful actress and he was at the top of his game in real estate. For both of us, like so many others, much of our identity was tied into our work, money and how much success we experienced. At this point, Alan was consistently feeling pretty good about himself. In my case, one minute I was on top of the world regularly earning hundreds of thousands of dollars, with press everywhere; and the next moment I could be out of work on the unemployment line, counting my change for gas and begging my agent for a general interview with any casting director he could find.

Alan had been seeing one girl, Sheryl, for two years. She was beautiful and known especially for her perfect body and long luscious hair. After the age of fourteen, I obviously could never compete for the best hair trophy. For both of these reasons, I always felt envious of Sheryl's attributes.

At the same time, she was a woman's woman (very important to me) and a genuine person with a good heart, who had to overcome many challenges in her life, so I both respected and liked her.

Through the years Alan knew nothing of my hair loss issues, nor did Sheryl. I would never let either of them get that close. But whenever we saw each other we were cheerful and loving. We had a good social relationship. From the beginning, Alan and I had chemistry and we were both Jewish, which was important to him. I always felt he wished we were dating but the timing was never right. One and a half years after he and Sheryl broke up and it was clear there were no residual feelings, Alan and I starting seeing each other romantically. It wasn't until our 7th or 8th date that I told him about my Alopecia condition.

Like most men, (and people in general) he had never heard of this condition and got a little frightened. I assured him that it was not contagious and that he wouldn't die from kissing me. It's amazing to me that there are some people who because they are unfamiliar with Alopecia, will go to that level of fear. Now that you know this can happen, the best approach with this type of reaction is to first, not allow yourself to take it personally. Understand that it's not 'you'; it's the condition they are unfamiliar with. Try to come from a calm place while using a little patience to educate the person and you will both experience an opening of mind and heart that will result in a good connection.

Over the next month he seemed to be more comfortable with it. Our connection was pretty good, our humor immense and our lovemaking superb. However, my wig drove me nuts during and after sex. Since there were no books available on any of this at that time, nor was anyone even talking about hair loss, I hadn't figured out how to be intimate with my wig on. I slept in the one that I had been romping around in, which was obviously now sweaty and incredibly itchy and uncomfortable. But as always, I would grin and bear it. I really never asked him how he felt about my condition,for fear of bringing attention to it.

Also, on a deeper level, I didn't want to tarnish the emotional high I was on. Our communication seemed to grow and overall Alan was a definite contender. As the weeks went on, so did the relationship.

Alan was into playing sports and wanted (expected) his girlfriend to be active with him. This raised one of my biggest fears – perspiration in public. Alan was an avid golfer and he knew I had considered going pro, so one of my greatest concerns was that one day, he would ask me to join him and another couple to play a round of golf. Heat and wind were not my friends, so this caused me constant anxiety.

In deciding to control the only things I could: my perspective, thoughts and feelings, I chose to stay in the *present* with each moment and not project into the future – something so many women do.

On only our second date, I had already picked out my perfect wedding decor!

I am much better with this now however, sometimes projecting the future creeps up on me; I affectionately refer to that as 'Future-ing" and have to remind myself or my honey does, to stay present in the moment. Thank you, Eckhart Tolle...

It had been about 2 ½ months. All was going well until one evening before going out, I noticed Alan seemed a bit more serious and quieter than usual. I asked if he had a bad day and he quickly responded, "No."

Sex, Wigs and Whispers

The drive to the restaurant was uncomfortably quiet and my internal alarm was ringing loud, driving me nuts. My gut had rarely failed me and I always (and still do) want to know what is going on, in the moment. His choice of restaurants was always lovely, the table predictably in the perfect location in the room; all so he could get a clear view of the attractive clientele and of course – so the attractive clientele could get a clear view of him. He needed to see and be seen. Even though he was more relaxed after a glass of wine, our connection was clearly off. Finally he said, "Listen Amy, you know I care about you; we've been friends a long time, and...umm, well you know, I... umm... well – I'm a hair guy. I mean you know me, you know my taste in women."

He began to ramble on...

"Just think about it; all the women I've dated have had fabulous long hair. I just have to tell you that I'm having a hard time with this hair thing. I've tried, but I just can't get past it. I'm sorry. I guess I'm just a superficial guy."

I felt like a spear had just pierced right through my heart. Electro-Shocked, would be a gross understatement of how I was feeling in that moment. I tried to remember to breathe and keep calm. Thankfully, after many years of therapy and working on myself via self-empowerment courses, books, along with my spiritual home, the Agape International Spiritual Center, I had become very clear on my own self-worth.

I responded, "Well, then I guess you're not the guy for me; because the guy that I will end up with will be far deeper than hair. He not only will be able to see past this unfortunate condition, but his focus will be on my heart and soul; who I am as a woman, his partner and his best friend. He will certainly be more interested in what we are to each other, rather than what I look like.

But it's obvious that's not something you can relate to. That's okay, you're a good guy; just a little fucked up. Now if you'll excuse me, I have someone fabulous waiting for me at home – me. I'll take a cab home."

And so I got up and sashayed off, while he continued to sit there, eat and people watch. So predictable; I thought 'how boring' and most of all, how sad.

The next time I saw Alan was five years later, at a phenomenal party thrown by a mutual friend, who to this day has one of the most unusual and striking homes I have ever seen. The grand foyer area made me feel like I was in an old Hollywood movie, replete with all the romance of Clark Gable and Vivienne Leigh.

The long and winding stairway added to the ambiance. Each large bedroom had its own fireplace, with a luscious sitting area connected to his and her bathrooms. They were all so well stocked from televisions to makeup, that you could live in them. The party was filled with Hollywood's most beautiful. I was certain the women hadn't eaten for a month or at the very least, were majorly bulimic to fit into their incredibly sexy gowns. All I could think of was, '*OMG! I have never seen so many perfect bodies and thin legs in one room!*'

It was catered with my favorite party foods: mounds of fresh large, tiger shrimp, lobster. and Bulgarian Osetra caviar. It was all so incredible that I just wanted to eat it with a spoon – which I did while no one was looking. *Tee hee.* I wondered if there was a security camera somewhere that caught me on tape doing that, because when I ran into the host a few months later he had the strangest vibe! As if he knew a secret. I wasn't sure if he really knew about my hair or worse – witnessed my caviar binge?! Oh well, the way I looked at it, at least the caviar didn't go to waste. I weighed myself the next day thinking how the hell I could

Sex, Wigs and Whispers

have gained six pounds overnight! I was holding so much water I looked like a blowfish!

Alan was at the party with his new wife; an attractive blonde woman who unfortunately was so manufactured, that whatever natural beauty she'd had was gone. Her attitude was very affected and insincere; she seemed more interested in showing off her six-carat diamond wedding ring and looking at her image in every mirrored surface, than actually having a conversation with anyone – including Alan or my date and I.

We stopped to chat. All I could think was, Self-involved and Superficial; Alan had found his perfect reflection. So, in a strange way I was happy for him. At the same time a wave of sadness came over me that he ended up with someone like that, instead of someone with better qualities or for that matter, me. Then I quickly remembered the tears I had shed and shared with my friends, after that last dinner with him. It was weeks before he called me to check in or see how I was doing after our abrupt break-up. When he finally did call, his only lame excuse for not calling sooner was that he just didn't know what to say. I found my strength and moved to the other side of the party.

Five years later, Alan and I saw each other again at a Christmas party. I was with my boyfriend, Jerry. It was a formal affair and I went all-out, purchasing a stunning French, red-velvet bustier, with a matching long, flowing, sexy silk skirt that draped behind me as I walked, adorned with a hand-embroidered matching red velvet shawl. This striking red was drop dead fabulous! One of my make-up artists gave me a most dramatic look accompanied by my splurging for a new long premium European human hair wig done with a deep sexy wave. I was feeling beautiful and hot.

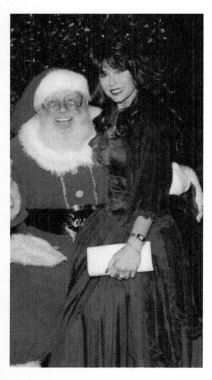

Alan was short; so when I introduced him to Jerry at 6' 3", my towering boyfriend (who knew the backstage about Alan) we were both 'Kvelling' inside.

*In Jewish, Kvelling means overwhelmed with joy; proud, to rejoice.

Yep, I was lovin' this moment! Alan was intimidated by Jerry and acted disinterested. Also, at that time he was not on the upswing professionally as he had been. His multi-million dollar mansion, once famous for the best parties in town, was now a small, rented condo and his expensive Mercedes was now a Honda. Of course, his wife was nowhere in sight.

Later that evening, when Jerry went to the bathroom Alan came up to me and said,

"You look so beautiful. I've often thought about you over the years with great regret about the way things ended with us. You know Amy, leaving you was one of the biggest mistakes of my life. I've grown so much since then. I would give anything to take it all back and start over with you. How serious are you with this guy?"

I happily responded with, "Well actually, we've been living together for three years; so I'd say pretty serious. And, although I appreciate your kind words, I must tell you that from what I've witnessed this evening – the way you acted towards Jerry, the women you're chasing at this party, your need to be seen

Sex, Wigs and Whispers

and heard, you seem to be as superficial as you always were. I want to be upfront with you though. When we were together, I was deeply in love with you. That night at the restaurant was one most difficult evenings that I have ever experienced. I cried for days afterwards. But because of how disrespectfully you treated me and how painful it was, it forced me to learn to stay secure in who I am. And that's helped me in every part of my life, including finding a deep man like Jerry. Plus, I've learned never to go back, only forward. I really do wish you all the best. Take care."

I took a breath and strutted away like a fanned-out peacock. And with no doubts or regrets, knew I had just given one of the best monologues of my life!

I'm happy to report that I recently bumped into Alan and we have rekindled our friendship. He is more conscious and humble now – I am too. Still single, he is much less concerned with his own needs and more compassionate of others. Alan gave me an incredible gift that night in the restaurant. One of the greatest 'reality checks' I have ever had in my life. And I passed with flying colors. When he 'assaulted me' with his own fears about my Alopecia, I was able to stand there, secure in my own worth and in my own greatness.

You will too…

AFFIRMATION

When I just take a moment to check in with my heart, and not my head, I will always be led in the perfect direction.

PART

4

Finally Ready

Smile – It's A Girl's Best Friend

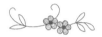

*"Life is 10% of what happens to me
and 90% of how I react to it."*

John Maxwell

'The best defense is a good offense' – We've heard it our whole lives, because it's true.

A Smile and Laughter is your best offense. Especially when fear, doubt, anxiety and uncertainty begin to fill you... SMILE!

I've said it many times throughout this book and anything worth learning is worth repeating *'What we think we create.'* What follows is a story that was definitely a first for me; and what a learning experience it turned out to be.

It was a typical summer day in Manhattan; ninety-five degrees, with ninety-five percent humidity; worse because I had been running around the city in this heat all day. The bus was packed like sardines, and all of us were in our own personal sweatbox. You get the picture. Sitting on the bus, I tried to sneak a quick look of my hair in the window but people blocked my view. Heat is a difficult issue while wearing wigs; (until you learn how to not make it one) so I had an aversion, bordering on a deep-seated fear of perspiration. Perspiration for me, is like nails on a chalkboard. Straining to catch a glimpse of myself in the window, I noticed a magnificent guy had wandered into the bus. He was the kind of guy that everyone, men and women alike, look at—a 6'4" Adonis, with green eyes (I'm always a sucker for those), and a body that made you wish 'take me now.'

I thought: *"OMG! Keep walkin' ...just a little bit further!*

I had recently been through a harsh breakup and this was the first week I felt ready to get out there again and there he was; my first top 'contender.' There was little doubt the universe had put him on the bus for me.

It took him forever to walk down the aisle, but when he finally came closer to my section, he was as gorgeous and hot up close as he was from a distance.

Sex, Wigs and Whispers

He stood directly in front of me, giving me *a most wonderful view.* Also, offering up to his towering 6'4" frame was a perfect view of the top of my head!

Oh No, can he see my wig?!

Fortunately, just then an elderly handicapped woman needed a seat; so I leaped up and let her take mine. That changed the configuration of things so that now, instead of Mr. Adonis looking at the top of my head, I was standing right beside my 'future husband.' I tried to play it cool when he looked at me, at the same time hoping that he would exit the bus with me, giving us a chance to get a substantial conversation going. All the while, standing on the bus, the legendary New York City potholes kept throwing us into one another. His voice, as inviting as his hot body, apologized each time he bumped into me, giving me an opportunity to gaze into his penetrating, sea-green eyes. *I imagined how green our children's eyes would be.* All of a sudden, we hit a huge hole and crashed right into each other! At first I was caught off-guard,

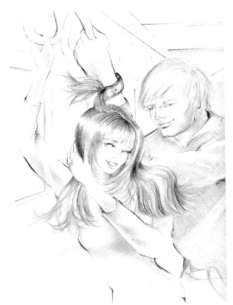

elated, until I felt his watch tangled in my wig.

I freaked!

"OMG he's gonna' take Missy with him! (All my wigs have names.)

Suddenly I acted like my own "real hair" was being pulled. Wanting to unhook us, he kept tugging his wrist backwards, forcing my head to jerk back.

I kept pulling my head forward to keep it steady, while shrewdly and firmly holding my wig down as inconspicuously as I could, trying not to panic. Before I knew it, I started laughing to make light of it and said, "Whoa hold on; let me do this my way okay – my hair – she's very sensitive."

He laughed, thinking I was kidding. Smiling, I said, "No seriously!"

He laughed again, thinking I was funny and cute. *Little did he know...*

A moment like this had never happened to me before and looking back, I was struck that after being without my own hair for so long, how innate the wig had actually become that it was automatic; it was like I was pulling my *own*, real hair, and since I truly felt that, so did he. The next five to ten seconds seemed like an eternity, jostling from forward and back, wrestling with my hair and his watch, keeping my wig in place and smiling throughout it all. Finally, after much struggling, my hair and his watch were separated. There was that moment when anxiety and fear were rushing through my blood stream setting it at an all-time high. And it's okay that this happened; it's absolutely normal. There's not a person who hasn't experienced that level of anxiety, sometime in their life.

We exited together and he asked me to join him for coffee to make up for the episode. Of course I jumped at his offer. At first I was exhilarated, but then the usual fear came up; the same old rhetoric that played in my head for years,

"I wonder if he can handle it?" or *"I bet he has a thousand girls with gorgeous hair – why would he want a bald one!"*

Sex, Wigs and Whispers

I quickly dismissed those thoughts and sat down. Just as I had imagined, he was sweet, funny, absolutely charming and sexy as hell... and recently separated, which I considered to be sort of available. However, "sort of" is like being half pregnant. You either are or you're not! And the recently separated men that I have experienced are rarely ever fully available, because they are still working through a lot of the issues that got them separated. So, the first women they get involved with after their separation are usually a pit stop en route to the one they end up with.

Although a hopeless romantic, after all the heartache I had just gone through with my ex-boyfriend, I swore, "No more repeat performances." I wanted someone who was emotionally and physically available the next time around. Since it was clear there was no future here, it was likely I probably would not be speaking with Mr. Adonis anytime soon. Feeling confident at having just handled a devastating situation so well, I decided to do something I had never done before; ask someone I barely knew if he was aware that I was wearing a wig?

"You're kidding right?"

"No seriously," I said, and proceeded to give him the Readers Digest version of my life with Alopecia. I purposely interrogated him; "Did you have any idea when my hair got caught on to your watch?"

"Absolutely not!" He responded, "Can I feel it?"

Wow! A complete stranger. This was certainly a day of firsts. *'Hmm – what the hell – got nothing to lose – go for it Ames'* and I put my hand over his (keeping me in control) and placed our hands on my head, allowing him to feel the wig.

"Amaaazing – I would never have guessed! You are so beautiful; really beautiful."

My insecurity flared up and I thought *'he's just saying that, trying to make me feel better.'* I immediately dismissed it, took a breath and then continued to explain that all of this was a first for me. He was being real. We both were. Genuinely sensitive, kind and supportive, he complimented me on my strength and I complimented him on his depth.

We never saw each other again – and never needed to. His gift to me was not being my mate, but giving me a profound learning experience that would forever transform my life. And just maybe he'll see this book and know how grateful I was for our brief encounter.

TIP: PERSPIRATION

The first secret is purchasing a lightweight, breathable wig.

As I always say, "Hold your wig up to the light. If you can see through it – you can breathe through it."

If you can't see through it, there is too much hair in that area of the piece. However, at the same time, there is a happy medium. You still need enough hair so it's not looking like bald spots in a certain place, especially at the top and crown. To achieve the most authentic look, you want the appearance of a part to be present, which should usually be 1/4" in width. 1/2" can look too wide with most wigs. It really depends on the type of look you want to attain. Again it's your choice.

It's a bit of a learning curve, but in a short amount of time you'll get to learn the difference.

Sex, Wigs and Whispers

If you find your wig tape releasing and your wig moving, just press down on the tape and see if it adheres any better to your skin. If not, run into the nearest bathroom, take off your wig, remove the used wig tape, clean your head with a little water, skin toner or witch hazel and pat your head dry. Then replace the tape back onto your wig and off you go.

TIP: BELIEVE

Stay centered and calm. People believe what you tell them and if your piece is your real hair to you, then it will be to them. Remember, you can fake it until you really believe it. Not giving in to your nerves and staying calm, smiling and laughter will help you here too. As I have repeatedly said throughout this book, it's usually our own insecurity and our own actions that give away our secret. The easiest thing to do is just go with the flow and don't overreact. The truth is, what we project and what we believe it to be is what translates to people. Thus, if your piece is 'your real hair,' everyone will believe it's your real hair. PERIOD.

Remember, the best defense is a good offense and nothing beats a genuine smile and sincere laughter that comes from knowing, you're just fine, as you are.

AFFIRMATION

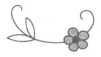

I have great communication skills when it comes to my hair loss. I'm in control and have the power over what happens in my life. My heart always guides me to the best way to approach any situation.

Smile - It's a Girl's Best Friend

On the Job

Stand and be counted or
lie down and be walked on.

Anonymous

iving with hair loss and all of the emotions that accompany it, can present a challenging environment for the hair loss sufferer as well as the people surrounding her. A client contacted me with a story about being called in for a meeting with her boss for her 6 months' review.

Her boss started out with, "Caryn, I brought you in to discuss your recent work progress. For the most part, you've been punctual and have tracked your clients well. However, your sales seem to have diminished a bit compared to last year. And I think I know why. You see, what I'm most concerned about is your personal presentation."

"What? I'm not sure what you mean by that sir."

"Well, you know that much of the sale has to do with one's personal presentation as well," the boss continued. "I've noticed that you have been looking a little unkempt lately – with your hair."

She was mortified.

"Can you do something about your bald spot? It's disturbing and may be taking away from your closing abilities."

I was furious that someone would be so insensitive and felt terrible for her.

Unfortunately she was not strong enough and didn't have the tools or the perspective from this book where she *could've* said to him:

"Oh, thank you. I was unaware of that. I'll make sure to work that in," with a smile of course, cool as a cucumber and walk out with her dignity.

Sex, Wigs and Whispers

She could have said: "Really – I appreciate you sharing this with me, I'm sure it wasn't easy for you to bring this up. The truth is that I have been dealing with a bit of hair loss due to a thyroid imbalance and I am taking care of it. However, even though I have been proactive I was unaware it was having this effect on my work. I will be more fully aware and focus more diligently on my work as this job and the company are so important to me."

Having at least one co-worker with whom you can trust and confide in that will be there to support you in times when your anxiety or fear may come up is very helpful.

If there is no one available, then make sure you are a phone-call away from your "go-to person"; someone you can depend on to center you.

Together, Caryn and I worked through both the emotional issues that were preventing her from accepting her hair loss and the steps we needed to make to help her find the right hair loss solution. We decided that based on her hectic schedule, dealing with a top piece would be too difficult for her as she would be consumed with making sure it was correctly placed onto her existing hair and would become a work distraction for her. We choose the Water Wig™ full cap design; it was a more simple process for her that requires less maintenance, as it returns to its original shape after washing.

Since many of us are concerned about the placement of our wig or hair piece, it helps to carry a small mirror to check your piece which can give you peace of mind. However, be careful not to obsess. This does beg the question:

How involved are we with our hair loss? Are we simply in denial and in not dealing with it, allowing it to affect us in ways we are unaware of?

If this sounds like you – ENOUGH – hair loss is not easy – but you can still look and feel beautiful with so many tools available to you now. It takes you making the decision to step into this positive perception or, continuing to sit there while you allow your life to unfold in ways that do not serve you. It's your call. If you are having difficulty, it's for you that I wrote this book; to help you move past the problems and live more freely.

You will find it's very true that with people in general and at work, especially in the area of sales, much of how people react to you has to do with your *own* confidence level. If your hair loss is affecting you at a self-confidence level – then let's do something about it. You don't need to have this condition take over your life to the extent of losing your job; due to either not having the knowledge of how to change it or the tools to work with the situation. No More excuses. Making the decision to move forward and be proactive about your life with hair loss is far easier than you *currently* may think...

If you have a small bald spot – go to your dermatologist and see if the cortisone shots, or maybe another new treatment is available for you. CreatedHair has been working with different hair growth products that have shown good success. Just contact me at: Book@createdhair.com and we can discuss other options.

You may only need a Top Piece, commonly known as a "Topper," a small hair piece that attaches to your existing hair with glue, small clips or tape. When a Topper is made or matched correctly with your color and style, it will add a beautiful layer to your already existing hair in the most discreet way. With a good one, you will not be able to see where your hair stops and the Topper begins.

The secret to attaining this result takes the following:

1) Getting a piece that fits your head correctly.

2) Making sure you match your curl to your real hair; If you have curly hair and suddenly wear a topper that is straight... how do you think that will look? Pretty obvious right?

3) Styling the piece in such a way that it blends evenly with your hair.

4) Making sure you match your style correctly. Toppers are available in many lengths starting at 4" and can be made as long as 24". But the more usual order is for 8-14" inches in length.

5) Matching your color correctly; Due to the fact that if you're dying your real hair it rarely keeps its color very long, there are two ways of doing this.

   a) Purchase a ready-made piece or have a piece custom-made as close to your own color as possible. If the piece is slightly lighter or darker in color, it will give the look of having put in highlights or lowlights into your hair.

   b) Purchase a piece close to your color and have your colorist match your real hair to the color of the piece.

6) Make sure to match your own hair texture as closely as possible. Ready-made pieces can be more of challenge in making this part work compared to a custom made piece made to match all that is needed for discretion. However, not all of us have the finances to do this. There are very good ready-made human hair pieces on the market which can be dyed and permed to your specifications. You just need to make sure the quality of the hair will hold up against the type of process you will be using on it,

i.e., processed blonde hair is difficult to perm, to color, and has a tendency of turning green when dyed. Virgin hair rarely will have this reaction. There are really pretty synthetic pieces that come in a variety of styles and colors with fabulous highlights and lowlights that you should be able to find one that works.

If you are at a point where there is too much hair loss to cover with a topper then it's time for a beautiful wig.

As I've mentioned previously in this book, it's important to keep a few things in mind when looking for hair pieces:

One of the most important secrets to making any wig or hair piece work is getting one which shows the part. "Monofilament" top pieces and wigs have a special material which is translucent at the top and shows your actual hair color along the roots of the hair. This special part of the cap creates the "illusion" of your skin at the root which adds to the realism of piece.

Make sure whatever you choose is lightweight. You don't want a heavy thing on your head 8-10 hours a day that you can't wait to rip-off when you get home!

Always look at the color of the piece in natural light only, not indoors. You may think your bathroom light is perfect, but the only light you can truly trust to get the proper color hue is in natural light. I always take my clients outdoors with a mirror and it's amazing how different some colors can look.

I remember the time a co-worker inquired about my hair. I was new to wigs and still hadn't found the right style for myself. He was a bit nosy and enjoyed being in everyone's business. When he had the nerve to ask me in that snide manner of his,

Sex, Wigs and Whispers

"Who did your hair today?" I told him, *"Oh please, does Macy's tell Bloomingdales?"*

Meaning – do both these famous stores share each other's trade secrets? He was stumped and laughed it off.

Other times, when he asked about my "color," but I knew he was really hinting at my wearing a wig, in a cruder mood I've responded with, *"Now, are you serious asking me that? That's like asking me if my cuffs match my collar! Get real."* (That immediately stopped him in his tracks.)

Just remember, you don't owe anyone an explanation. If you decide to answer their inquiry then do so on *your* terms – when you are ready to. Being prepared with your "elevator speech" to assist you with a quick response that you're comfortable with is always good to have in your back pocket.

AFFIRMATION

I can handle any spontaneous moments with my hair.
I am in control and know exactly how to respond with
confidence and absolute assurance of my own I Am.

"Toppers" (Top pieces)

Medium Topper 10-12 inches

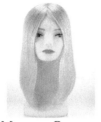

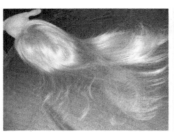

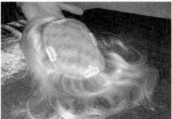

Medium Blonde Topper

French top/Straight

Topper Base

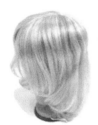

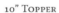

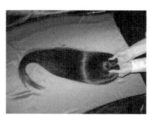

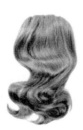

10" Topper

Monofilament Part

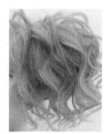

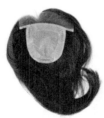

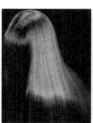

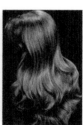

Curly

Lace Front

Medium Brown w/ Large "S" Wave

16" Brown Straight

16" Brown Wavy

Sex, Wigs and Whispers

Intimacy is Ageless

IT'S NEVER TOO LATE TO BE SEXY

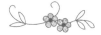

"Love doesn't make the world go 'round,
love is what makes the ride worthwhile."

Elizabeth Browning

Sophie Rubinstein was eighty-one years old. It was one of those overcast days and I was pretty pooped from the week. All I wanted to do was lie down in a warm house on a comfy couch placed right in front of the TV, with a big bowl of popcorn and a box of black licorice; when all of a sudden the phone rang with a very loud Brooklyneese voice on the other end that began yelling:

"ELLO, ELLO ? IS THIS AMY GIBSON?"

"Yes, it is."

"CAN YOU HEAR ME?" the annoying voice demanded.

"Yes, I can hear you. How can I help you?" I confirmed.

"LISTEN, MY NAME IS SOPHIE, AND I AM EIGHTY-ONE YEARS OLD; I LOST MY HUSBAND 2 YEARS AGO AND AFTER TEN YEARS I BEAT THIS CANCER THING! I'M READY TO GO OUT THERE AGAIN! I WANT TO LEARN HOW TO DATE WITH THIS THING ON MY HEAD AND I HEAR YOU'RE THE GIRL TO TEACH ME. CAN YOU HEEEAR ME?"

"Yes, yes I can hear you. Okay, um, let me get this straight; you want to learn intimacy with your wig on; am I correct?"

"YOU GOT IT. DEAR; I MAY BE OLD BUT I AM CERTAINLY NOT DEAD!"

I loved her already!

For years, women have flown in from all over the world to take part in my Pearl Program. In half a day together, I teach them a variety of intimacy tips that they can take with them to help

Sex, Wigs and Whispers

them go through their intimate moments successfully. Sophie scheduled her appointment for the Pearl Program.

I hate to admit it, but at first I was a bit uncomfortable as I had never coached anyone over sixty five. After a lot of small talk, I finally got up the nerve to ask her,

"So how intimate do you want to get, Sophie?"

Her immediate response, "Everything; I want to feel again, be alive, in every way. After all the money I spent on therapy, I deserve it!" *I immediately knew we were going to have a fabulous time.*

There are two key factors to successful intimacy: being ready and being willing. Sophie was both. However, until our meeting, it never occurred to her that she could actually control the situation – tell her new man *if* and *when* she wanted and *how* she wanted to about wearing a wig – meaning that she could *choose* the circumstances. This is not unusual. Sophie, like so many other women, just assumed that a man would know she was wearing a wig and therefore had hair loss. Embarrassed, shy, for some reason feeling less than another woman, giving up her power to him – not taking control – this is how most women are. We began our journey together.

As boisterous and strong as Sophie came across, she actually was much more sensitive than she let on. She was more concerned about a man finding out about her hair loss before she had a chance to get control of it, or possibly tell him herself, then she was about sharing her body with a new person – even though she had only shared her bed with the same man for fifty-eight years. So we worked on it; sharing many of the tips you'll find in this book.

We went for long walks on the beach and she learned how to deal with wind and perspiration. We went over how to approach a man she found attractive – because in her dating days, women were far less assertive. We reviewed kissing with her wig on, and how to avoid his hands in her hair during several sexual scenarios. However, she seemed to be fixated on her years of talent that earned her the nickname as 'the BJ queen.' I must admit, I even learned a thing or two! We explored the more serious moments of when and how to tell him about wearing hair, which to my surprise, appeared to be difficult for such a tough woman. But, she worked through it or as she often put it 'Got over it.'

We worked on manifestation by exploring the deepest levels of what it would feel like to be in love again; feel that wonderful high again. What it would feel like to have a new man to wake up to and cook breakfast for; and what it would be like to go on a long, romantic walk again, arm-in-arm; and how it would be to allow herself to cuddle him under the moonlight. She was a joy to work with and I never laughed so hard with a client.

A wise woman, our elderly bring a sense of deep insight like none other that can only come with years of life experience. They have found no-nonsense ways to look at life that is both inspirational and humorous; and at times, have also left me a bit confused while my young heart and mind grasped the full scope of their brilliance. I've always had a pet peeve with the way these wonderful human beings, our wise ones who have helped build this country, are treated and oftentimes forgotten about.

In our time together one thing became crystal clear; although generations may have altered how lovers are together, sex and intimacy never really changes. Like riding a bike; if you've done

Sex, Wigs and Whispers

it once, you'll stay up on that bike again. Passion, with the right motivation, attraction and inspiration, can be ignited again. You never lose it. Like many people, I have always worried about my libido disappearing as I age. And certainly with menopause, I have had my challenges with this. We could talk about that for days (hormones, stress and nutrition play a large part!). But right now let's stay on point.

The work Sophie and I did together was enlightening and freeing for her, opening up possibilities that would alter the course of her life and making it possible for her to have a chance at a new life. Until we met, she wasn't sure that would be possible ever again.

This is common and more the norm than not. Even the wisest and strongest of women face this 'personal' challenge when dealing with hair loss. Intimacy and sex with someone new? Oh, let's face it! Even with our long term lovers, it's full of unknowns that can be emotional and scary, preventing many women (and men) in the best of circumstances from even going there. Hair loss for a woman, even those that appear to breeze through the experience, is anything but normal; so intimacy, sex and passion can suffer, leaving a void in someone's life. We are all Sophie and no matter what, deserve to be touched and loved.

TIP:

Don't be afraid; you are no different in your sexual essence just because you lack your hair. Sex is captured as an energy, just as much as it can be in a look. However, I find the energy to be far more powerful than the look. Get in touch with that essence again.

Remember what it was like when you first felt really sexual with that special person. Remove all judgment and just for a moment, forget about it; put it aside and keep focusing on that incredibly hot and sexy feeling. Think about when you looked good in that bra, or how great it felt laying there in the nude, while your partner just devoured you with his eyes. The feeling that you had when you knew you were exciting him, just by that look that you gave him. You had him – that power.

Remember again and again, how that relief felt when you had an incredible orgasm with that person? How sexy you felt afterwards, how sensual, how proud, how womanly you felt. The way you walked when you got up out of bed. That, ladies, is energy. There is nothing more powerful in that moment.

Meeting Sophie was both an inspiration and a relief. It always amazes me, yet I know it's true, that whatever we want in our lives is possible depending on how we think; it's just all in our minds. I was reminded of the pure truth of this once again, with Sophie. She decided to fill that void in her life; and nothing was going to stop her. And that was it.

Shortly after we had completed our sessions Sophie met someone. At a hair loss support group of all places! He is bald and "God gifted" as she put it (I later learned that meant well-endowed and a great lover). Within eight weeks she moved to the Midwest with him and found a new meaning to her life. I never heard from her again; but I know she's doing just fine. People like Sophie always are – because they choose their own reality and make their own happiness.

Sophie, if you're reading this you'll see the impact you had on my life, and the support you have been in my quest to help many other women transform their lives. From all of them and myself, thank you.

Sex, Wigs and Whispers

AFFIRMATION

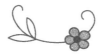

I can feel my body again. I am feeling more alive every day.

I am beautiful, I feel sooo sexy.

I can take a deep breath,
and literally feel that raw sexy energy
running through my body;
in my groin, my stomach, my throat, and my lips.

Sex, Wigs and Whispers

Oooh! Broaching The Subject

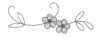

"Take the first step in faith.
You don't have to see the whole staircase.
Just take the first step."

Martin Luther King, Jr.

As always, the decision whether or not to tell him is up to you.

Here are a few different approaches that I've used in broaching the subject of hair loss which have worked most of the time:

1. CONTROL AND CALM

"Listen, if we're going to be friends, it's got to be based on honesty. I need to tell you something that's been on my mind. I have been dealing with a condition that has resulted in losing my hair and it's been stressful trying to be someone else for you when I am with you. It may or may not grow back. It very well could... I didn't know how you would react so it's taken me a little bit of time before I felt comfortable enough in sharing my secret."

Remember, staying calm and in control works; it's only when our reaction becomes abnormal that people sense something is off, curiosity sets in and that strange uncomfortable dance usually follows. The easiest thing to do is just go with the flow and not react. Just respond to him, not too strongly. Most of the time, if you are ready to discuss this and are in control of your emotions, the words fall into place just fine. Please believe me when I tell you it's easier than you think. It's all in the approach.

2. UPBEAT AND BOLD...

"Honey, let me ask you something; on a scale from 1-5, what physical quality would you say is most important to you? Are you into...say... legs? Hair, tushie, face? Some men are into eyes, etc."

Put the word hair in the middle of your sentence and do NOT stop or pause when you say the word – just follow with your question. WAIT for his answer. Regardless of how long that moment may feel. MEN NEED TIME TO PROCESS. Don't be

Sex, Wigs and Whispers

thrown off, just continue as planned. Most of the time men say their preference and it will usually include hair. If he doesn't mention it and it doesn't come up in conversation, you may feel the need to inquire further with,

"So uh, how important is hair to you?"

WAIT for his answer. Those of us who are uncomfortable with the waiting have a habit of answering the question for them. So just give him the time he needs to respond. If he responds with

"Hair is definitely on the top of my list." DON'T FREAK – just stay calm and say

"Hmmm, interesting – I would have taken you for an eye guy or leg man."

Translation: GET HIM OFF THE SUBJECT OF YOUR HAIR! Stay in your power ladies – think sexy... _not_ OMG I have none, Now What!

The good thing is that you have your answer, this guy's into hair. Okay, so always make sure _yours_ looks great when you see him. This does not mean that he won't fall in love with you because you have none. On the contrary, it means you have some inside track now, as to what makes him tick – which is a good thing; because now, you just have to work with that until he gets to know _you_ well enough so the hair won't mean as much. He'll be more connected with _who_ you are and the hair will no longer take precedence. Now it will be your heart, your sense of wit and charm, that will be at the top of his list. But first, you need to give him time to get to know those wonderful things about you. In the meantime, make sure your hair looks luscious and smells nice.... :)

If he responds with never mentioning that hair is important – you may also just leave it alone, don't bring attention to it. Just enjoy the moment.

3. Fun and Flirtatious

A bit of humor always works for me. However to use this one, you must have your emotions and your 'story' in tact without any emotion attached or it won't work correctly.

Be upbeat, flirtatious and stay away from being serious when you say this. At the same time be genuine.

"So… do you like _my_ hair?

Of course they'll say yes. Then reply all in one sentence, with a BIG SMILE,

"Oh thank you", (Take a beat) as you run our hands slowly through you hair;

> "Do you want it? You can have it – because I don't have any. DON'T STOP – That's not a problem is it? (Big Smile) TAKE A BEAT – Great!"

Common responses are:

> "Why no, of course not, I care about you." (Let this one soak in) or

> "Well, you need to give me a minute to digest this."

My solution for this one is,

> "Go ahead. I totally understand. This is a bit different than what you're probably used to."

And then – give him the time to think about it, without freaking out or being afraid that he's going to run. Being rejected is what most of us are so afraid of. If you stay calm, he'll stay calm and be open to the communication. As long as you stay true to yourself

Sex, Wigs and Whispers

and your feelings, you will both be fine. However, you don't have to sit there and remain uncomfortable. If you find he's taking too long to react, make light of it with an obvious look at your watch, followed by:

"OK – so, you're good...? No heart attack on the rise?"

As if giving him a moment to review, then try laughing it off. This will help keep it light.

Now that you've dropped the bomb, immediately move on as you normally would in a conversation, like nothing had just happened. Move on to something completely different – something positive and upbeat. Again, <u>show NO emotion</u>. "So have you seen any good movies lately?"

It will be up to you as to how involved you want to get into this subject matter with him. Obviously you can't drop a bomb like this and not expect a reaction. Anyone would have questions and want to know what happened, so be prepared to answer. If you're requesting honesty from a partner and you're sensing that he's uncomfortable with your last response, should he want to know more, be prepared to expand on your explanation because he deserves to know.

Obviously, on your terms and ONLY if you're ready.

At this point it is critical you stay centered. Tell your story, <u>without the drama.</u> This is usually the part that will freak a man out. Rehearsing in the mirror or with a friend helps before broaching the subject.

Most of us have endured pain, suffering and just plain drama throughout this process; but for now, save this part of your story for your girlfriends. You can share all of what you've been through with your man, when you are both in control of your feelings. Don't be fooled; this is a big deal for him and you. Give sharing your secret the respect it deserves and wait.

However, if he wants to discuss this further and you <u>don't</u> want to get into it any deeper, with EASE, say...

> "Why don't we talk about this later? I'll fill you in on all the nitty gritty, but right now let's be here together." The key here, is to let it be and truly <u>move on</u> with your evening. Don't harp on it. Try to enjoy and focus on your time together.

But trust me, 99% of the time, anyone will want more information – and being prepared helps you be in control and keep your power.

4. CURIOUS

If he's curious about your hair and begins to ask about it and you're not ready, try this for a diversion;

> "My hair – ah – that's a boring subject. Let's talk about something more interesting!"

And <u>move on</u> to just that – something more interesting. He may back down which is fine and... he may not. He may ask again. In this case, be aware not to completely ignore his need to know. Remember, he does have a right to know the person he is dating. Respect his wishes and mention that you'll take the time to address it later on. However, do this on <u>your</u> time table – not his.

5. PLAYFUL, FLIRTY, SEXY

This has always worked for me when I have not only been ready to tell him, but when there has been enough intimacy to take it to the next step and be more physical together.

In a so soft playful way – not serious at all here ladies, ask him,

> "So, you think about it; in your life have you found yourself drawn to more blondes, brunettes or redheads? What about women with dark, sultry black hair?"

WAIT for his answer. If he says, "Why are you asking?"

Just tell him, "I'm curious." Some men will tell you, while others may say:

> "I don't know, it doesn't really matter to me, I like all women. It's more about the connection" (I like those…)

Or they may say;

> "I don't know, I've never thought about it."

Then you can try one of these, which has never led me astray,

> "Well, what if I told you I could be anyone you want me to be? How fun would that be?"

If he says, "What do you mean?" I like to play and say,

> "Well, just use your imagination… what if I could look any way you wanted me to? I can be Audrey, the blonde bombshell one night; or I can show up as Tara, the sultry, long haired brunette, with nothing on but thigh high boots under my fabulous leather trench coat… Just think about it, you never need to have an affair, because all you would have to do is make a request for the evening and lo and behold, she would appear at your door. You can never tell who you're going to get."

*This particular one should be said only with the utmost of confidence and playfulness. If not, it will come off insecure and you'll ruin the entire intention and the moment. At this juncture, say what is most comfortable for you and your heart. Say a lot or say nothing; it's your choice. If not, it's okay. You can stop right here and leave him alone with his imagination.

Ooh! Broaching the Subject

6. Not Ready to Share; Intimacy and Sex…

I'm always a fan of intimacy and sex; But, if you're not quite ready to tell him and want to avoid him touching or even getting close to your hair, tell him,

> "Oh listen, I had these extensions put in and my head's a little sensitive. So I'd appreciate it if you don't touch my hair."

If he gets nosey and has the nerve to inquire further about the extensions, just stay calm and play-it-off with,

> "Seriously? You must be kidding. That's a little too personal. Down Boy!"

So as to avoid that weird moment, quickly but subtly move on to another subject.

There are many more How To's about this and other 'Hot' topics in the **Nookie Time** section of the book. Now go Have Fun!

AFFIRMATION

I make perfect choices for myself. I'm in control and I know exactly what I need to do and what to say in any situation that arises.

When Considering Intimacy

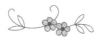

"Attitude Is A Little Thing
That Makes A Big Difference."

Winston Churchill

Intimacy is a lot of things, including sex, but not exclusive to sexual activity. No matter what kind of intimacy you are looking for, this chapter will help you. I know we have gone over this, but there are two points we've discussed thus far that are imperative to remember:

1) The way you present your information to someone is exactly how that person is going to interpret it, and sets the foundation for their reaction.

2) Being in control of your emotions is critical. It's helpful if you remember to share your condition without all the drama it's brought you. If you are emotional, the response you will receive will be as well. If you freak out, he'll freak out. He becomes your mirror. It's a lot to ask of someone to not only hear you, but handle all their emotions and yours – simultaneously.

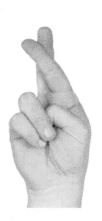

There were times I would keep myself calm by doing what my dear friend, wonderful therapist and KPFK radio host Nita Vallens, suggested. Whenever I'm feeling out of control or unsure, whatever the reason, I crisscross my middle finger over my forefinger under the table. It somehow immediately breaks the emotional cycle or attachment. This small technique has worked great for me for fifteen years, and still does to this very day.

The way I see it you have four choices:

1) Don't expose yourself or say anything about hair, touching your hair, etc. Avoid any conversation that could lead to the subject of hair or physical touch. This can be stressful but at times it's the best thing to do if you're attracted to your date and don't have a handle on your hair loss yet.

Sex, Wigs and Whispers

2) Lie and literally bluff your way through the moment; specifics of how to do this are in the chapter "Ooh! Broaching the Subject." However, if you do choose to bluff, make sure your story stays consistent.

3) Always have other people around you and your date, until you are more comfortable. Don't put yourself in a position of being alone with your date.

4) Keep the friendship on a phone call basis until you're ready to see him in person.

In my many years of dealing with my own hair loss, there were men in my life who had their own issues with it, which created interesting lessons for me. When my article in People Magazine hit the stands I had an ex-boyfriend (operative word being "ex") call me whom I had never told about my condition, and the conversation went like this:

"Hi Amy, it's Barry."

"Barry, to what do I owe this unexpected pleasure?"

"Well, I saw you in **People** and I wanted to congratulate you. I think what you're doing for women and children is just so beautiful."

I said, "Thank you."

"Amy, there's something I want to say; can I tell you how I really feel?"

Barry was intense. He was addicted to EST, a personal growth course given many years ago by Warner Erhard. Erhard's approach was to empower people and help them transform themselves. And "how he felt" always prefaced anything Barry would say.

"Okay Barry, what is it?"

"Well, I have to tell you, I feel a bit betrayed."

"WHAT?"

I took a breath.

"Be-trayyyed?!!?!?!??"

Another breath.

"Really... and why would that be?"

"Well, we dated on and off or two years, and I'm just surprised that you never told me about your hair issue."

I took a beat,

"Well, first of all Barry, when will you realize it's not always about you? Second, maybe I never felt safe enough to let you in that deep. And third, Wow, I just can't believe that after reading this article your first thought is about my not 'telling' you about my hair. After two years of dating, perhaps you should've said,

"OMG Amy, I had no idea what you've been living with. Are you okay?"

He was silent; I said,

"Barry, maybe I never trusted you enough to tell you. Maybe I knew you would have considered only your own feelings and what this did to *you*."

I waited for his response, and as he began his defensive answer, I quickly said, "Barry, can I ask a favor?"

"Sure, anything."

"Remember this tone." And I hung up.

TIP:

Well, by now I'm sure you get the gist; only tell your partner when you feel ready and secure. Not before. If they are so insecure that they do not want to wait for your comfort zone, then Move On.

AFFIRMATION

Not everyone can handle it... That's THEIR problem!

PART
5

The Nitty Gritty

Living a Full Life with Wigs

New Beginnings

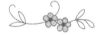

"When one door of happiness closes, another opens; but often we look so long at the closed door that we do not see the one that has been opened for us."

Helen Keller

There are no excuses for not enjoying life to the fullest. You can work out, go dancing, be intimate and have lunch with friends. Be as physical as you want; take a long bike ride, a yoga class, water ski, ice skate, go for it all! Life is certainly a journey. Living with wigs does not have to make it more difficult unless we decide that it is. Wearing a wig just makes life *different*. And sometimes that's a gift. **I know some of you are saying "How the hell can losing my hair be a gift?"**

In the beginning, I asked God many times, *"Why did this happen to me and what the hell am I supposed to now?"* I'd beg God, *"Please just return my hair to me and then everything would be back to the way it was. I could get back to being me again."* But what I soon realized was that I would never be the old me again. Losing my hair made me different, better, deeper, more intuitive and slowly I got my answers.

It took me getting to a place of acceptance with my hair loss; forcing myself out of the anger, depression and sadness, moving beyond feeling like a victim and instead, getting to a place of being grateful. My Mom's earlier words to me that I had previously resented would now echo in my head,

"Amy, what you don't realize, being so caught up in your hair loss, is that you're luckier than most."

I would answer,

"And how the hell is that!"

"Well God graced you with a beautiful face – you can walk, you can see – hear clearly – you are lucky enough to have two breasts – that's how. Let's be grateful for those things. We can replace the hair. Now let's move on already."

And she was right. The more grateful I became, the easier the process was to accept my new journey.

Sex, Wigs and Whispers

How you live your life wearing a wig all depends on your attitude. Is the wig a part of you, like your arms and legs and your real hair used to be? Or is your wig something detached from you, some foreign thing that you put on your head every day? The decision to accept, or not, is yours. It's all about your perspective; once again... it's up to you.

Granted, a wig is not your real hair. It does not grow from your scalp. Therefore it is different. But today there is a plethora of wonderful "alternative hair" to choose from that will make you feel as if it is your very own hair. These options weren't available to me when I first lost my hair. Now, in many cases, you can get a wig that comes very close to the look you once had. For many, your new 'do' can look even better. Many times I will say to my clients, *"So do you like your hair?"*

'It was okay,' is often the reply.

Well, why do you just want 'okay?' This is an opportunity for you to be anyone you want to be. You can have even better hair – a better look – a better style or color. Hell, let's be a Diva! Let's give you the same look with better hair. Let's just go for it!

Do not be afraid to live – to try new things and new looks. Who cares what anyone thinks! If you try it and it doesn't work, you can always change it back. That's why the world of wigs and extensions can be so wonderful. It offers you an incredible playground in which to explore all your personalities and fantasies. And it can be loads of fun with your partner to enhance your intimacy.

As I've mentioned previously, when I lost my hair and began my 'alternative hair' journey, nothing looked or felt right.

They all looked and felt so fake. Nothing came close to making me feel like *me*, there were many tears shed in every store I visited.

Living a Full Life with Wigs

I drove the sales people nuts, along with any friend who accompanied me. The truth is, it also had to do with the types of wigs I was choosing and my lack of experience wearing and styling them; but it had a great amount to do with me accepting my hair loss.

The day came when I stopped making excuses, stopped the anger, stopped blaming every wig designer and stylist I met with and embraced this new experience as one of hope. I decided to embrace this journey and create a fabulous new me. Suddenly, as soon as I made this decision, I was able to find beautiful wigs. This is a perfect example of what I refer to when I say it's all about choices. And just as instantly, everything seemed to fall into place. The synthetic wigs I found and had easily styled suddenly filled a great void in my life for those quick trips to the market. And the human wigs that I found really felt and looked exactly like my own hair. They were so well-made, that I immediately felt like 'the me' I was before losing my hair. There was no longer the need to be ashamed or hide; my hair loss was a fact I accepted. Having lost my hair is way of life now, and I still love exploring new options.

That's right ladies, now you can feel secure enough to allow yourself to ROLE PLAY! Go a little crazy!

TIP:

You want to keep the look as natural as possible but still give yourself an improved look with a little more hair – operative word being "little." Whether you're wearing extensions or a wig, your intention is to match your normal look, usually by adding no more than 20% hair to the existing thinner hair. By adding only 15-20%, most people will wonder what's different about you and ask why you look so good!

Sex, Wigs and Whispers

They'll say,

"Is it your color? Did you lose weight?"

This is the desired result you want to attain. You never want them to say, "I love your new wig!" Most ladies prefer discretion so, if you care to share – then go for it – but only when you choose to. But if all the notice to your new improved style leaves you feeling awkward, don't feel you need to suddenly explain your new style. To me nothing could be more uncomfortable. Just offer a gracious,

"Thank you."

Before I went public with my hair loss, when someone used to comment on how great I looked, asking about my colorist, I'd say,

"I use someone who comes in from Europe – I can hardly get in to see her, she's so booked." Or "it's a brand from Europe – I can never remember the name."

Always careful to respond with a cool calm demeanor, of course.

How __you__ feel is the real difference and fortunately, with insights from this book, you can be in full control of your mind and your emotions.

Over my fifteen years of working with women's hair loss, I've surmised that usually 48 -78 hours after losing their hair, most women completely forget their exact color or style and it usually takes looking at photos to be reminded again. I was in such trauma, that for me, it took just 48 hours to completely forget my exact color.

If you are about to enter into treatment or notice hair loss, this makes it even more important to keep photos of yourself with your favorite styles to continue looking your best. Keep a small but good sample of your hair taken from the front, sides, top and back.

Keep these samples separate in marked bags; so if you do need to, you can recreate your look.

Most women are off by at least half a hue or more. At CreatedHair.com and Salons, we'll try several colors until we find the just the right one that makes the client "pop"; meaning a color which compliments both the client's eyes and complexion, thus giving them their best look. Women tend to get used to their same look and they never consider other color possibilities. Most stylists/colorists avoid suggesting something different because it's met with so much resistance; so they just keep doing the same color. Then, there are those women who just don't know the difference so they play it safe. Playing it safe in life drives me nuts. It's claustrophobic.

AFFIRMATION

My hair not does define me.
My heart and mind do.

Sex, Wigs and Whispers

The Art of Hugging

"Our life is measured by the risks we take"

Ali from
The Bachelor, Season 14

There are many types of Hugs:

The good 'ole family hug is the kind where someone takes you in their arms and gives you a strong Bear Hold that you couldn't break free from to save your life. Generally, you'll find that this person is unaware that they're pulling your hair off, which in your case, might mean literally.

Then there's the OOOOOH hug – the one that goes on forever that you *want* to relax into… Instead, you cringe; scared this person is going to touch your hair. Or worse yet – take your hair with them!

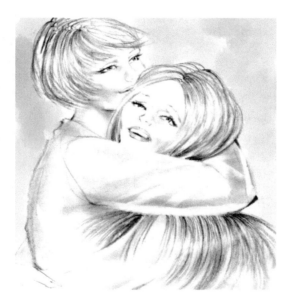

Relax – I know it's the last thing you're comfortable doing right now. But do it anyway, because the calmer you are in these moments the more success you will have.

Sex, Wigs and Whispers

In both these examples, if you find that someone is hugging you and they begin to sway – sway with them. If your hair is tangled in his arm – go with it, and gently offer with a smile,

"OOPS! You got my hair!" and laugh it off.

If they begin to rub your head lovingly or abruptly, try,

"Oh not my hair honey! I just got it done.'"

Men usually make a crack or two, in an attempt to be funny. The truth is that men get a little uncomfortable around hair issues, and just don't know what to say, so they laugh. Remember what I've said before; continue on as if nothing happened.

If you know you're going to be in the environment of several hugs, it helps to lightly braid your hair to one side. This lessons the chance of your hair getting caught in someone else's arm pit!

AFFIRMATION

I act my way into a new way of thinking, rather than think myself into a new way of acting.

Sex, Wigs and Whispers

Hair Petting

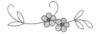

"The pessimist complains about the wind; the optimist expects it to change, the realist adjusts the sails."

William Arthur Ward

What makes someone want to touch your hair?

People are drawn to three things aesthetically – light, texture, and color. Think about it: How many times has someone approached you after getting your hair done when it's nice and shiny? That's because they're drawn to the light, texture and color of what they believe is your hair – most of the time we never think much of it. Those of us who are 'wearing hair' need to remember that nothing has changed for the people around us – they still want to touch our hair if it looks shiny and soft. So, when someone 'pets 'your hair, don't shy way. Remember, it's a compliment.

There are plenty of women with real hair who choose not to have it touched so, there's no reason for you to feel strange if you prefer not to have your hair touched, just because you don't have real hair. You have the same rights as any woman with natural hair. You still have the right to say NO to anyone, at anytime, anywhere. When it comes to touching your body – No – does not mean maybe. It means NO. Nothing has changed.

TIP:

With that in mind, when someone you know reaches over to touch your hair, don't bolt. If you're comfortable, stay calm and allow them to feel it. For a moment. I would subtly move my head away from their hand, as if to say, "Thanks, that's sweet."

If someone you don't know unexpectedly touches your hair, by all means say "Excuse me, but I would prefer it if you did not touch my hair." When they complement you on your beautiful hair, look them straight in the eye just as you normally would when someone pays you a compliment and say 'Thank you' with a smile.

Sometimes, you may get a compliment on your sudden 'great look,' but they won't know what exactly it is that looks different, just that it's pretty or better. A good wig should have this result. You can always say, "Oh, yes, thank you. I put in a little color." (Tee hee!)

AFFIRMATION

No – I won't if I don't want to.
No – You can't if I don't want you to.
No – I do not need to explain myself to you.

Sex, Wigs and Whispers

Hair Pulling

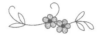

Nobody gets everything in this life.
You decide your priorities and
make your choices.

Donald E. Westlak

I had a client who called me frantically from a family outing. She was appalled when her brother-in-law thought it would be entertaining and funny to play with her hair and then suddenly gave it a strong tug. He had no idea he was pulling her wig that was clipped in – it ripped my client's hair. She panicked and didn't know what to do. Everyone was watching – her entire family and some friends did not know her secret; something she had kept private and sacred. I was grateful she thought to call me so I could help her. It gave me the opportunity to explore this issue further for the book. How would you handle this? After reading this book, hopefully you will do the following:

TIP:

1) *If someone reaches for a tug – say "Ouch" as if it's your own hair. And then, "Please don't tug, my hair is very sensitive."*

2) *If you are caught off guard when this happens, remember that people will only react to what you react to. If you fluff it off, they will do the same. If you make a big deal and draw more attention to yourself, then you will reap the consequences of that.*

3) *Avoid letting it get to the point of pulling on your hair to begin with. Use the many techniques discussed to get his attention off you and back onto him. Because really, he was doing this for himself anyway. So getting him to focus on himself will not be difficult.*

4) *Kindly tell him – in a cute way – that you prefer no one touch your gorgeous hair!*

5) *Do not feel guilty or uncomfortable in saying this; be empowered.*

6) *Lastly, do all of this with a smile – and stay as cool as a cucumber!*

Sex, Wigs and Whispers

AFFIRMATION

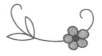

*I am gently, compassionate and
understanding towards myself.*

The Big Screen

KEEPING YOUR SECRET... SECRET
AND YOUR DATE CLOSE

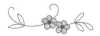

"The only people who never tumble are those who never mount the high wire."

Oprah Winfrey

So, he decides he wants to be romantic and take you to a movie; here are a few things that can happen when watching the big screen:

1) He puts his arm around you and mistakenly rests on your hair.

2) Someone walking behind your chair mistakenly leans on your hair or their bag catches onto your hair and pulls it.

3) He goes to kiss you. He first puts his hand behind the nape of your neck and is about to feel the bottom of your wig. Oh Nooooo!

If your date and his arm are suddenly resting on your hair or someone walking behind your chair mistakenly leans or catches onto your hair and pulls it, as my astute sister once told me, *"Don't trip potato chip."*

TIP 1:

Try to remember that over time, your wig will become part of you. If your piece is secured with tape, clips or bobby pins just react as you would if your real hair were being 'sat' upon or pulled. Sometimes I've said in an easy voice "Ohh, can you lift your arm? You're on my hair, Honey." Then afterwards, thank your date for removing it.

Or, "Oops, you've got my hair" and continue as anyone with real hair would – they move on. Don't dwell. We have a way of lingering ladies – we can get OCD, which gives us away. For anyone who does this, it's critical to be in control. And remember, once again – most people are too caught up in themselves to even notice.

Sex, Wigs and Whispers

If it's not secured and your piece has moved, quickly look down at the floor as if you're looking for something that may have dropped and subtly put your piece back into place. Or, you can pretend you have to tie your shoe and fix it while down there. Do anything that gets your hair/wig out of their direct eye. Then, get your tushie to the ladies room and fix 'Mildred' so she's secure.

The main intention here is to get his attention off your hair and onto somewhere else.

If you choose to wear a full wig here is some helpful insight...

When I first began to date prior to getting a handle on my hair loss and how to live with a wig, one of my greatest fears was when my date would reach his hand behind the nape of my neck and possibly discover my wig. Most women find this a terrifying challenge. And worse, many I have spoken to over the years stopped having an active social life and dating, because they didn't know how to navigate this intimate situation with a wig on, and still keep their secret.

If he slowly reaches his hand behind your neck and does the usual slow 'neck rub' you have two choices...

1. *Act totally self-conscious and move abruptly, which will most likely create an uncomfortable moment.*

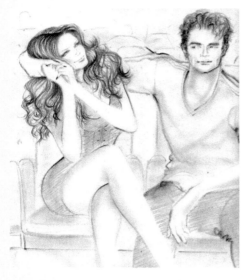

Or...

2. Calmly take your hand and move it slowly until it barely rests on top of his. Now, move your face and nestle into his hand. It's when the hand is free and may go a bit higher on the nape, which is where the base of the cap sits, that it can become an issue. Just don't let him go there. Period.

This is very endearing, and has always worked for me. Additionally, your eyes can help as well. Give a soft sweet look and watch him melt.

If you're sitting, and he's someone 'new', the knee is a safe destination to place his hand.

You can be playful provided you have that kind of a relationship. And then by all means, use your imagination; place that hand on where his body is calling for...

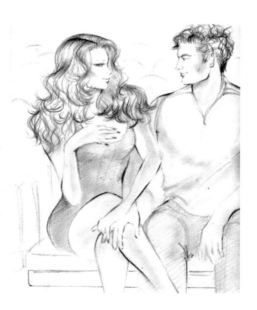

Sex, Wigs and Whispers

AFFIRMATION

I am ready to date with my wig on.
I know that as long as I stay true to my heart,
and respect my inner voice,
there is nothing I can't handle.
I am fully prepared and now free from all fear and worry.

Preparing For The "Unexpected"

*"If opportunity does not knock,
build a door."*

Milton Berle

IF YOUR DATE SHOWS UP IN A CONVERTIBLE...

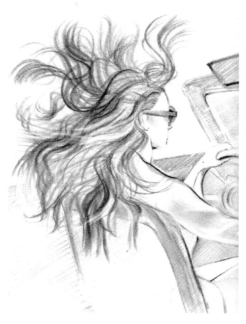

TIP:

You have two choices:

1) *Roll up a small tightly fitted hat or headband, and place it in your bag. Whenever you feel comfortable, nonchalantly take out the hat and place it on your head. Most of the time, men have gotten a kick out of my being 'prepared' even though they never knew my secret.*

2) *Listen to your heart. If you're uncomfortable about this it's absolutely fine to gently ask him to put the top up. If he says "Oh, I was hoping to smell the fresh air," etc. Respond with – "Me too, but I just spent so much time making myself beautiful for you." They'll always put the top up!*

Sex, Wigs and Whispers

However, if you do come across a date that is determined to have it down – then you continue to honor yourself and say, "I understand, however I prefer to have it up!" Stick to you guns! You'll feel more powerful and in control if you do, and ultimately, more comfortable and confident.

And remember ladies; MANY women with natural hair would say exactly what's I told you to say above. This is less about your piece, and more about what makes <u>you</u> comfortable.

AFFIRMATION

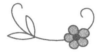

I am not afraid to honor myself and my needs.
I no longer need anyone else's approval
to make me feel accepted.
I lovingly accept myself,
which is much more powerful
than anyone else's approval of me.

The Jacuzzi

*"One important key to success is self-confidence.
An important key to self-confidence is preparation."*

Arthur Ashe

There are a few things that will help if you can bring them or if it's unexpected, you should be able to find them. Women by nature are intuitive and good snoopers when we need to be. *Oh come on, you know what I'm talk'n about. We've all been there! You're gonna' tell me you Never looked in your host's bathroom cabinet – we all have!*

Isabella was one of my wonderful clients who had just turned 21 and was dealing with Treatable Hodgkin's Lymphoma. Oddly enough, young girls afflicted with Treatable Hodgkin's is something I have seen more this year than any other year I've been in business. Isabella had the spirit of a falcon and was extremely funny. She was young and spunky and her outspoken nature reminded me of my own. However, Isabella was still in the midst of finding her sexuality, so her hormones were raging. Her humor and quick wit gave her the ability to say things that were of a serious nature without alienating anyone.

Like me, Isabella was a true Sagittarius; and if you're Sag, you know exactly what I'm talking about! At least people know what they're getting into when they meet us; Sagittarians are notoriously blunt, have no tact, very little diplomacy and rarely think before we speak. You never have to wonder where we're at. It's all over our faces. OY! The trouble I have gotten myself into – speaking my mind! It gets exhausting!

Isabella was beautiful, with long, thick brown hair. When we met she was emotional and frightened and knew she was about to lose all her hair; it would fall out in just days from chemotherapy treatment. With a rockin' body, she was hot and sexual, with long legs, perky boobs and was an accomplished athlete. Then she got sick.

It's interesting; I find younger women and children more easily walk through the hair loss process than most adults.

Isabella knew she was lucky to have the means for great treatment and doctors. However, like most of us, no one explained the process of hair loss to her; so in addition to feeling fragile and vulnerable, she was confused about what to expect. She was committed to continuing her active life with friends and dating, but had no idea how the heck she could do this with a wig on! After all, how many 21 year olds do you know who wear a wig?! And most women, of any age, are just lost. Nothing prepares them. But at 21, it's an even greater challenge. However as with everything, wigs just takes patience and trust – and practice.

One night the phone rang at 10 pm. I picked it up. It was Isabella with an emergency. She was at a party and everyone was having fun... in the Jacuzzi; she didn't know what to do. As wonderful a time as this sounded, it also presented a greater issue for Isabella; there hadn't been enough time before she went out, to go home and get her matching inexpensive synthetic piece we had previously purchased for this sort of surprise. We had gone over the instructions of how to do the 'quick change' many times so she would have it down pat. Instead, Isabella found herself facing a group of young twenty year olds, shouting for her to join them in the hot tub! With ONLY her expensive Russian piece that she had just purchased from my studio.

I told her she had a few choices: "OKAY, let's breathe for a moment and we'll figure this out."

TIP 1:

Twist your hair and pin it up with a large barrette to hold the hair in a ponytail. Isabella had a lace front piece which was very natural looking and had no wig edges. However, if you're not wearing a lace front piece, bring the first row of hair from the bang forward. If the bang is long, move to either side or tuck behind your ear.

The Jacuzzi - Expect the Unexpected

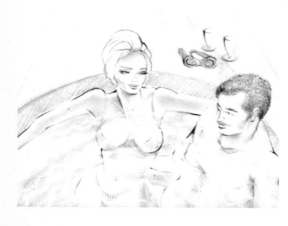

Let the sides of the piece hang down a little; this will hide the edges of the wig.

After that, I told her she could relax a little.

TIP 2:

For me, taking a towel and twisting it into a turban has always worked great! The towel keeps the hair from getting into the water. That's of course unless you go further down into the Jacuzzi water; then the piece will get wet. If that happens when you come up from the water, pull the hair out of your piece as instructed above.

TIP 3:

Get a small white towel. Step into the Jacuzzi and twist the towel tightly; then quickly wrap it around your neck – propping you up a bit while resting against the side of the Jacuzzi. You can pull

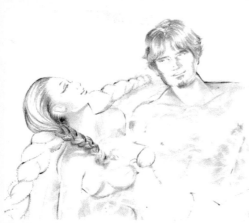

your hair around and braid it. This will keep your hair at the nape of the neck dry, or at least dryer than if you were without it. The rest of your braid may get wet; but that will dry in time, no worries! And you will look cute in the interim.

Sex, Wigs and Whispers

TIP 4:

If you are not wearing a lace front wig, apply the same technique as you did when wet; by pulling your bangs forward and down, with the sides going in a forward direction in order to hide the outer edges of the wig. With a lace front, the hair can go back and you won't see the hairline; but it's more secure to just pull the hair forward at the front and sides to avoid any unnecessary snafus...

TIP 5:

You can also open the towel and place it behind you on the cement; so when you lean back, your hair is spread out on the towel. This keeps it off the wet cement. You can always say you don't want to rest your hair on the dirty cement. And remember ladies – add a little lipstick or gloss – it always looks sexy!

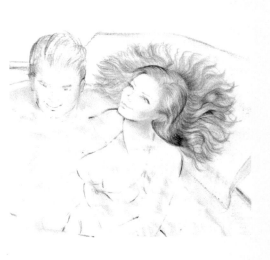

REVIEW – HANDY REMINDERS:

- An extra synthetic wig to interchange with your human hair wig.
- A small towel that is large enough to twist under your neck, but not too bulky.
- Another small towel to place on the outside of the Jacuzzi on the cement.
- A large barrette to hold your hair in a ponytail.
- Bobby pins.
- A small mirror always comes in handy.

Since human hair drags a bit in when wet, just let it be. DO NOT SCRUB IT DRY WITH A TOWEL AS YOU WOULD YOUR REAL HAIR or it will tangle the entire wig! After patting the wig dry, shake it a bit to get any existing water out of the piece. Unless you have good conditioner on the piece, try not to brush it when wet. You can use a wide-tooth comb to slowly untangle the piece.

Isabella was much more in control after our talk and it all worked great. She had a fabulous night. The towel worked perfectly until she got dunked right into the Jacuzzi! But because she had gone through my *Pearl Program* Isabella didn't panic; instead, she knew exactly what to do and did not overreact. She went with the flow of the moment and had a blast! The Pearl Program showed her how to hide the frontal hairline and calmly excuse herself to find a bathroom; there, she could pat the piece dry and carefully comb it out. And because she took the time to honor her needs, she was able to step out, take care of business and get right back into the party with ease and confidence. With NO ONE the wiser! And you can do the same.

AFFIRMATION

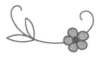

I take the time I need to take care of me.
I am strong enough to overcome any fear in my life.
I breathe in confidence and breathe out all fear.
I choose to dissolve all fears that darken my being.

Blowing Away

*"You never change things by fighting the
existing reality. To change something,
build a new model that makes the
existing model obsolete."*

R. Buckminster Fuller

Something as simple as walking with your date can be stressful for the wig wearer if you're walking into the wind. As I mentioned earlier in "Honoring Yourself," opening a restaurant door and walking into a building through a moving

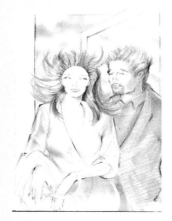

door can be additional concerns as this can force the front hair of the piece up and backward – thus exposing the edge of your piece.

You can use this tip for walking on the beach, or whenever you may find yourself in a gust of unexpected wind.

TIP 1: THE "TUCK"

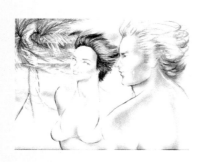

Just like I did with Steve when we walked into the restaurant against a gust of wind, lower your head slightly and tuck your chin down a bit – but just a bit – or you'll look like you have a crick in your neck! Remember, subtlety is key when dealing with hair loss.

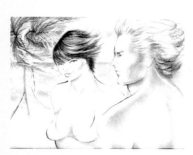

The wind will push the top of your hair downward, instead of blowing directly into your face and lifting the bangs backwards.

Sex, Wigs and Whispers

Investing in a good hair system can make all the difference in creating a strong level of comfort. Lace front pieces might work well, but keep in mind that if you plan on wearing a lace front piece every day, the lace has a tendency to tear and get worn out. Depending how hard you are on your pieces may result in the lace needing to be replaced approximately every 5-6 months.

However, you can camouflage the front edge of wig by styling baby hair into the wig. (refer to Styling section).

Over time my piece has become part of me, and with a little practice all these techniques worked better and better as I got more comfortable with both my hair, and the process.

TIP 2: THE HEADBAND:

This is always a great accessory to have with you in the car or your bag. In the past it has been a lifesaver against the wind. It's the reason it is included in the ResQ Bag™.

A headband can come with bang hair already in the band. If they don't have bangs you can create the look yourself, if the headband is made in a way that will support you changing the look a bit. Here are a few ways to work with headbands with hair:

2) If you want to use your own hair with the headband; after placing the headband on your head, pull all the hair back from the very front of your hair, draw out a very small amount of hair and bring them forward to stick out in front, offering a more authentic look. You can also pull out a small amount of your own hair from the sides and use this with the headband as well. This is what we refer to as giving an illusion of Baby Hair. (Again, see Glossary and Styling Section)

3) You can also bring more hair forward to create a heavier bang.

4) If you are without hair and desire a more authentic look, you can purchase a weft of hair that can be sewn underneath the front part of the headband to create bangs as well as the sides to create a more realistic look of sideburns. For further information on this, write me with your questions and contact information to: Book@CreatedHair.com and we'll will be happy to address your inquiry.

5) If you have no hair and want to secure the headband, place a small piece of wig tape at the front, sides, or nape of the inside of headband to adhere to the scalp. I suggest sewing a piece of thin polyurethane (available at CreatedHair.com) or a small piece of silk material (1x1") to the inside of the headband where you will be placing the tape. This will easily grab on to the tape without stretching the material of headband.

Careful: If you do have some hair and choose to use the tape in places that you may shave or you may have no hair, it's most important that when removing the headband to be careful not catch any existing hair onto the tape and rip the hair.

If you have enough hair for a small clip to catch onto then by all means sew one onto the inside of your headband. To prevent the clip from peeking through the headband material and giving away your secret, I suggest sewing a small smooth piece of silk. Since you want to careful not to use a piece too thin, you may need to double it before sewing it onto the headband where you will be placing the clip(s).

Sex, Wigs and Whispers

AFFIRMATION

As I challenge my fears,
I become more strengthened & empowered.

Dive In

"The only thing worse than being
a late bloomer, is being a never bloomer.
It's never too late."

Darren Lacroix

One of the most common questions I am asked is "How do I deal with my wig in and out of the water and still keep it on while looking great and feeling sexy? The concern is a good one because we want to be interacting with our friends and dates as we always have and/or would like to. You can participate in all water sports and it's easier than you think! There are several ways to assist you in working this out with materials that help keep the wig on and prevent it from lifting up or off the head. It will all be with ease... you'll see. After we're through... you'll be dipping for days!

As a sports fanatic, I was forced to find ways to deal with my wig while swimming, water skiing, and even water slides... I refused to stop doing things I loved!

TIP 1:

Making sure to use wig clips attached to your piece or two-sided wig tape is an essential tool to have with you if you plan on doing water sports or being active with your wig on where perspiration is present. (More on this in chapter "Working Out")

TIP 2:

One sneak tip is to always carry a travel size spritz bottle full of of wig conditioner. Quickly and nonchalantly, lightly spray the piece when you get out of the water. This will help immediately de-tangle the piece and avoid possibly pulling out any unnecessary hair, leaving it straight and clean looking when it's time to brush it. Keep in mind that you must use the conditioner sparingly on your piece or it will get too sticky and need constant washing. Too much washing will compromise the quality of the hair. Some of the color may release from the piece as well, thus shortening the overall life of the piece.

Sex, Wigs and Whispers

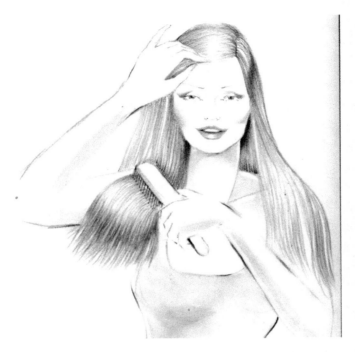

When brushing, remember to always hold down the front of the piece or the bang delicately with your thumb and forefinger or you may pull it off. (And we certainly can't have that) You can do this with some style, as illustrated.

AFFIRMATION

I, and only I decide:
When, Where, and How I wear my hair.
I allow the real me to radiate out.

A Wild Ride

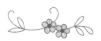

Twenty years from now you will be
more disappointed by the things
you didn't do than by the ones you did.
So throw off the bowlines.
Sail away from the safe harbor.
Catch the trade winds in your sails.
Explore. Dream. Discover.

Mark Twain

A woman contacted me who was hysterical because she was on a roller coaster ride with her grandson, when her wig suddenly flew off and was hanging on a tree! At first, I thought she was kidding; until I realized how truly upset she was. I asked her;

"So let me get this straight; when you left your house today did you know you were going to be at an amusement park? Didn't you realize you'd be going on rides with your grandson?

She muttered, "Yes."

"You didn't clip in or pin down your piece?"

She muttered, "No."

I continued, "And, you're at an amusement park in Florida and you're calling me in Los Angeles! How can I help you from here?"

Frantically she said, "My friend told me to call you and you'd know what I should do."

I felt terrible for her for so many reasons, starting with her grandson not knowing she wore a wig. After calming her down, we got proactive. First, she ran into the gift shop and purchased a cute bandanna; then, I went on the search for a wig store in her area, where she was able to get a new wig.

TIP:

It's all about being proactive and prepared ladies. Sitting in your situation and letting it fester doesn't do you (or anyone else) any good. Take actions to help yourself! On this crazy wig journey, prepare for the expected. The only way we can change our reality is making the choice to do just that, change.

If you're going to be active, for extra security, bring a hat or headband. And don't forget a few pieces of wig tape or wig clips!

Sex, Wigs and Whispers

AFFIRMATION

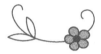

I know the appearance of things
does not always mean it is my reality.
It's just the appearance.
Life is temporary.
Change is always certain.
After all, our conversations will never take place
in the same way again.
I am staying in the knowing, instead of the fear.

Working Out

"Life is either a daring adventure
or nothing at all."

Helen Keller

What do you do when your man invites you to workout at the gym or outside?

Don't panic ladies… there is a way that really works.

I know right now you're thinking, "OMG – how the hell am I going to keep this thing on while jumping around at the gym? Won't it be too hot to work out in? And what if it falls off while running?"

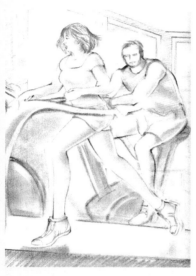

Working out with a date is great fun for most people, but for the wig wearer it can be hell, since most wigs get warmer with exercise causing heavy perspiration. *So being prepared is critical and is the difference between a miserable fear-based experience and a joyous, fun one. I know, that as long as you're prepared with what you need at your fingertips to make you look and feel like the 'old you' (pre-wig), everything is easier to maneuver.*

When I'm working out, if I look in the mirror and like what I see, I push harder. It's not about my goal weight or how toned and lean my body is. All that matters is how I feel about myself; if I'm feeling good, my workouts are great! Let's face it ladies, when we feel hot we work that much harder at getting even hotter!

Another thing I have gotten very clear about over time is that regardless of where my weight is at, usually if my hair rocks, I rock!

Now… here's one of the worst moments of my life which, after reading, you will diligently follow below and be prepared!

Sex, Wigs and Whispers

My LA gym was the Sports Club and I had it down to a precision change, like a race car driver in a pit stop. I would go into a stall, remove my dry wig from a plastic baggie and replace it with the wet one that I had just worked out in, clean my scalp, replace the wig tape, pop my dry one on in 2 minutes and be out. Only on this particular day, the only stall available was a handicap stall with a curtain, not a door. The locker room was packed. It had only been a short time since I lost all my hair and I was still in a bit of trauma over it while trying to continue living my life as normal as possible. My wig was drenched from my workout so I couldn't wait a minute longer. I thought *I got this; I'll run in really quick and get it done.*

No one had ever seen me without my hair; I was completely bald. In the midst of changing my wig in that stall without the door, out of nowhere a handicapped woman in a wheelchair came into the bathroom, and suddenly pulled the curtain to the side and started screaming at me, calling me every name in the book for using a handicapped stall.

I was mortified. Everyone was looking! I quickly threw my dry wig on which I'm sure was on backwards. I tried to apologize but she continued to scream at me while everyone stared. Completely humiliated, flustered and utterly horrified, I tried to grab my wet wig and all my accessories, but they kept falling everywhere.

I stuffed everything in my bag and ran out. I sat in my car for an hour and cried. I vowed that day that I would do two things:

1) I would create a wig that every woman could exercise in, swim in, shower with it still on, that would dry in its original style within minutes and most importantly, allow her to feel *normal*. I imagined myself in this process and

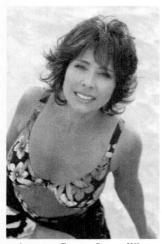

being able to put on my makeup next to every other woman in the dressing area while my wig dried naturally on my head just like their own real hair would and how wonderful that felt.

2) I would create a sexy, discreet bag that didn't look like an obvious wig bag so I could keep my secret, and

AMY IN CYBER SWIM WIG

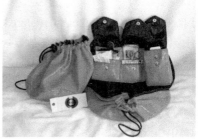

that would hold a wet or dry wig, extensions and all wig accessories needed in one convenient place. Then flashes of what just happened brought me back to reality.

Years later, the First Women's Swim Wig with Cyberhair® and the ResQ Bag™ were born.

Learn from my pain and humiliation and you'll always be ready to have a great workout experience.

TIP 1:

The ResQ Bag™ – The First and Only Carry-All Kit for Wigs and Extensions. Now you never need to be embarrassed by your hair loss again. The 2 piece ResQ Bag™ includes: a Mini ResQ Bag™ with a Patent Pending Design that is completely waterproof, which helps reduce any matting and frizzing of alternative hair and includes The 12 Care and Comfort Tools for any wig emergency.

Sex, Wigs and Whispers

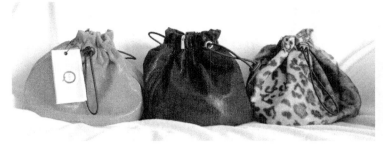

ResQ Bag™

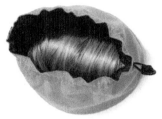

INSIDE YOU WILL FIND ALL YOUR GOODIES THAT ARE INCLUDED IN THE ResQ Bag™.

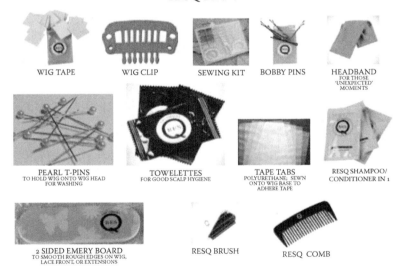

WIG TAPE

WIG CLIP

SEWING KIT

BOBBY PINS

HEADBAND
FOR THOSE
'UNEXPECTED'
MOMENTS

PEARL T-PINS
TO HOLD WIG ONTO WIG HEAD
FOR WASHING

TOWELETTES
FOR GOOD SCALP HYGIENE

TAPE TABS
POLYURETHANE; SEWN
ONTO WIG BASE TO
ADHERE TAPE

**RESQ SHAMPOO/
CONDITIONER IN 1**

2 SIDED EMERY BOARD
TO SMOOTH ROUGH EDGES ON WIG,
LACE FRONT, OR EXTENSIONS

RESQ BRUSH

RESQ COMB

ResQ Bag™ is a dream for anyone wearing a wig or extensions. It has everything you need at your fingertips.

TIP 2: Headband

Bring a headband to either hold your hair back off your face with just the bangs showing, or to place around your head to help keep the perspiration from running all over your face.

Another wonderful, comfortable product that has really come in handy for me is a headband with the synthetic hair attached directly to it. They are usually sold in one size, come in an array of colors and lengths and are available mostly with synthetic hair, but you can also find them in ready-made human hair. Although for the client looking to match their own look, I have personally designed them in human hair as well which is always fun. As I've mentioned in this book, if the headband has no bangs, sewing bang hair into the headband will add to a more natural look. I usually will sew baby hair onto the sides as well, giving it the illusion of real sideburns.

If your finances are a bit tight at the moment, and you need bangs, no worries. Just take one of your old synthetic wigs and measure one inch behind the front of the cap and cut straight across four to five inches. Having hair that is already attached to a base will be make it easier to sew on to your headband. Take the piece and attach it underneath the headband, cover and sew a soft piece of material so it won't itch your skin, and let the bangs hang forward. When I no longer had any my old wigs to pull from, I purchased the least expensive wig I could find and cut that one to fit my needs.

For Sideburns: remove the sideburns from your old piece as well in the same fashion and attach them again from underneath the headband material to the area where your normal sideburns would hit your face. Don't get frustrated, this just takes a little focus and proper measuring to make sure the hair is lined up correctly with where your own sideburns are or would be.

Sex, Wigs and Whispers

Most hair loss replacement centers will be able to do this, or feel free to email my office at Book@CreatedHair.com, and you can receive a quote for the cost of doing this for you.

TIP 3: WIG TAPE

If you use wig tape to keep your piece on, realize that most wig tape will have a tendency to loosen with perspiration; the solution is to always bring extra tape with you. Be careful when using red tape because it can be a little irritating to the skin on a daily basis. Water Wig™ tape, which can be purchased from CreatedHair.com, is strong and used for activities and swimming, as well as for those with heavy perspiration. There are several other tapes on the market, including lace tape (usually in blue) which also work well.

TIP 4: ADHERING YOUR WIG

If you have hair that appears sporadically and want to prevent the tape from sticking to your existing hair, take a little hair spray or water, and push your hair back away from the adhesive area, making sure to keep it dry before applying tape.

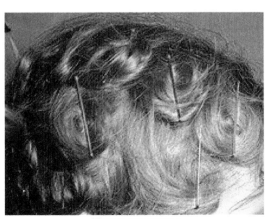

TIGHT PIN CURLS

If dealing with longer hair, you can also make small tight pin curls, and pin them above or away from where you are placing the tape. To do this, take small sections of your hair; roll the hair around your finger, and pin it to your existing hair.

If you want the front of the wig to be secure and do not wear your own hair, you can shave 1/10th" at the front and place the wig tape there.

Note: As with any adhesive, before applying, you first should check for any allergic reactions. Take a small strip of tape on your skin and wear it for 5-10 minutes. If you don't itch or have any swelling you're good to go. If you do have a reactive response, then consult your physician for further alternatives.

If using wig clips just make sure you have securely attached the clip to your hair. If you have thin hair try twisting a small section of hair for the wig clip to adhere to. Oftentimes this will hold the clip better. However, whenever using clips, make sure to be patient and remove your wig or extension carefully so as not to tear your hair.

TIP 5: Changing into your wig

- *Go into a stall in the ladies room – grab a few paper towels.*
- *Take your wig off.*
- *Wipe your head with either toner or witch hazel – a good wash of soap and water can work fine.*
- *Let your head dry for just a few seconds*
- *Remove tape from piece and replace with new tape.*
- *Wipe the inside of the wig with a paper towel to help lessen the amount of perspiration in the base fabric.*
- *If you have an extra piece with you, at the end of the workout follow these same steps and then change into your new piece. He'll never know...*

Sex, Wigs and Whispers

TIP 6: SCARF

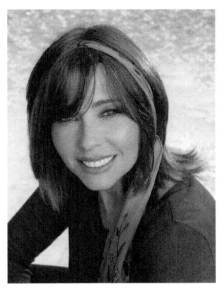

You can also do wonders with a scarf:

Wearing a scarf can work great especially if you add a sexy pair of earrings, and beautiful lipstick or gloss! Ladies, you can go without makeup... but never without lips! They frame the face and bring light to you.

To help you decide whether to work out with your man or not – first ask yourself this question:

How comfortable am I with this wig process before I agree?

Before you go on your workout date or consider intimacy... go over this checklist;

1) Do I have the right wig to exercise in?

2) How about the right "dry" wig to privately change into?

3) Do I have all my wig accessories?

4) Do I have a headband to keep my wig on and away from my face?

5) If your answer comforts you, then go for it. If not, you have two choices:

a. Refrain from going for just a bit longer until you can practice on your own at the gym, and then invite him over at at later time.

b. Make sure you have your tools and push yourself to go. It'll probably be worth it!

AFFIRMATION

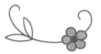

I have a total handle on how to live my life normally with a wig on. I no longer worry about any surprises that may arise, as I am fully prepared with what I need to feel secure and at peace.

Sex, Wigs and Whispers

Careful Not To Sizzle!

"What would you dare to dream
if you knew you wouldn't fail?

Brian Tracy

A Chef in the Kitchen

One of the most challenging things about entertaining is looking fab in your wig while cooking up a storm. There are two challenges: perspiration and burning your wig.

If I'm alone, I obviously will prepare dinner in my turban or a pretty scarf. However with company, I prefer to have my beautiful hair on.

TIP 1: Perspiration

Perspiration is difficult and wearing something to keep you cool will help with the added perspiration that happens in a kitchen. Either braiding your hair and pinning it up in a barrette or simply twisting your hair and clipping it up, will help keep the perspiration off your nape, an area that is most challenging and can quickly create frizz. Wearing a headband can also keep the perspiration away from the nape.

Sometimes I have worn a synthetic 'headband with hair' (discussed in the chapter "Working Out") that is close in style and color to the hair I have chosen to wear for my evening guests. Then after I am finished cooking, I'll excuse myself and quickly change into my good wig. No one ever caught on – again, proving that most people are consumed with the moment and not your hair.

TIP 2: Burning your Wig

A. *The most important thing to remember is that any type of hair burns quickly.*
   You need to be aware not to get too close to the heat or your hair will quickly sizzle.

Sex, Wigs and Whispers

If you're stirring a pot of sauce, stand back a bit and make sure you lean away from the heat when looking to see its progress. Don't put your head over the pot to get a whiff of the gorgeous aroma coming from your pasta sauce. Do this as far away from the pot and as quickly as possible. I prefer to dip a large spoon into the sauce, move away from the heat where I can taste and smell the sauce, thereby removing any chance of my hair turning to dust!

B. *If alone, remove your wig before reaching for the pan. If you're around people, ask someone else to remove the pan. If no one is available, then please don't place your head into the oven to grab the pan of salmon. (Yes – you guessed it – I have ruined many a piece. LOL) Keep your head as far away from the oven as possible while placing your hands in the oven and quickly grabbing the pot. You don't want the oven heat to escape too long and finding its way onto your quickly melting fiber.*

TIP 4: RESTAURANT / HEAT LAMP

Sitting by a restaurant heat lamp can be a disaster for us girls!

If you have the ability to choose your seat, make sure it's not directly under the lamp.

I try to stay as far away from the lamp as possible; however, if you're caught by surprise and placed under the lamp, sit there for a bit and then don't be afraid to check with your guest/guests before asking the restaurant to turn down the heat or off for that matter. If the other guests at the table prefer to have the heat on, ask to trade places with one of the guests on the opposite side of the table telling them you prefer to be a bit away from the heat.

Be Careful Not to Sizzle!

Again, honor your needs first. You paid a lot of money for your investment. Protect it regardless of the opinions of others.

AFFIRMATION

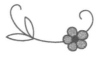

I am mindful of the hair that I wear when exposed to heat, and I calmly make appropriate choices to assure my needs.

PART

6

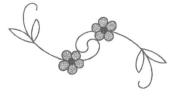

Nookie Time

Your Bed or Mine

*Before you say "There are no good men",
make sure you are a good woman.
Sometimes you attract the lifestyle you live.*

Ilovemylsi.com

PREPARATION

This ladies, is honoring yourself and owning your power.

What happens if you forgot something!

I'll never forget the time I had finally gotten to the emotional place of being intimate with someone and we planned the perfect evening....

We had been dating about nine weeks and my "boyfriend" *(of course, I was already daydreaming about our impending marriage)* was cooking a romantic dinner. I purchased an expensive human hair wig and had it styled to perfection. The cherry red on my nails matched my lingerie and sexy heels; also purchased earlier that day. To be frank, I truly felt like I was rockin'. At least *I* thought so – which is all that mattered.

When I arrived at my boyfriend's house it was obvious he had put enormous effort into preparing for our evening. It could have been in Hawaii. Lighting and flowers lined his long driveway; and the luscious scent followed me all the way to his doorstep. He gave his housekeeper the evening off so we had absolute privacy. The interior design of his home showed his talent for aesthetics. There were cobalt blue velvet curtains, matching sofas and red flowers bounced that off the reflection of the polished marble floors to perfection.

The coup de grace was that Mark was an incredible chef. He created a delicate and sensual meal with spectacular wine. Candles bathed the room in romantic ambiance.

We began watching a movie in his custom home theater and in time we started kissing. When he reached over to touch

Sex, Wigs and Whispers

my hair – I told him that I had gotten a perm earlier and my head was very sore; I asked him to please not touch my hair or head. As he knew what was waiting for him, it was easy to get him to comply.

Although his house was beautiful it had a strange layout. The living room and home theater were on the opposite side of the house from the bedroom. As we were moving into a more serious level of foreplay, we left kissing and moved onto unbuttoning my blouse; I took my cue and immediately excused myself to the bathroom. I was nervous so just the thought of finally getting to this point with him had me ultra-excited.

Everything I needed was packed, and I was fully prepared from mouthwash to protection. However, as I opened my purse I realized that my matching "thrasher wig" that I normally would change into to romp around in, was actually sitting in a bag back at my apartment. I did not want to ruin my expensive human hairpiece by sleeping or romping in it or get it matted from perspiration. Between my raging hormones and this hiccup, my heart was thumping so loud I had to throw cold water over my face just so I could think. Keeping in mind how much he loved my hair, my next thought was 'security' – I made sure to secure my wig with extra wig tape. I went back into the bedroom and just kept my hair out of the way by pushing it over to the side as much as possible. I knew the difficulty would arise when it was time to sleep. To lessen perspiration and keep it from tangling, I put my hair up into a comfortable bun, so the nape was the only thing touching the pillowcase.

Satin pillowcases are great for reducing hair static and I was sooo grateful he had chosen a satin bed set! This allowed me to keep my 'little lady' fresh.

Sleeping in a strange bed with a new person can be uncomfortable enough. My new wig was hot and itchy, which made for a sleepless night. I made it a point to rise quietly in the morning before him, so I could give my scalp the needed breather, brush through my piece and have it looking just like he remembered it a few hours earlier.

Luckily, all went well; but following this, was one of many reminders on how important it was for me to be organized and prepared whenever I went out. With Wig Intimacy, preparation is the means to success.

TIP 1: WRAPPING YOUR HAIR

Wrapping your hair is certainly one way to keep the hair under control while sleeping, and will prevent it from getting tangled and frizzy. This technique will also leave your hair smooth. I call it making the 'Big X'; mainly because that's what you're doing.

Divide your hair down the back vertically in half; take a small amount of hair from the right side, pull it across the back to the left side, and make sure it's flat when pinning it down. If your hair is long – make pin curls while keeping them as flat as possible.

Now, like a crisscross pattern, take a small amount of hair on the left side and pull it across the back to the right side; again make sure it's flat. Repeat going from side to side like an X until all your hair is tightly tucked in pins.

If you have curlier-styled hair, nightcaps and scarves are especially useful for reducing hair friction. If you plan on tying the scarf, you'll want to make sure that you tie the scarf in a way so that no hair gets caught in the knotting.

Sex, Wigs and Whispers

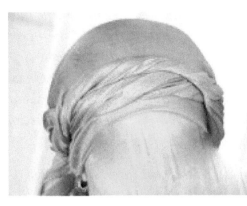

Many women find it simpler to wrap a scarf around the nape, then continue bringing it up around the forehead and back down to tie at the nape in order to avoid tangling the hair when tying the scarf. Just make sure you make that scarf look really cute! It's all about the vibe ladies... if not for him, do it for you!

It's okay to take the time you need to make sure you rock, feel hot, confident and ready to take your man (and you) to places he's never gone before. You may encounter the challenge of keeping your beautiful piece from getting ruined during repeated intimacy. Consider the price of a good wig and how much effort it takes to keep it in good condition and you'll want to find ways to extend its shelf life.

TIP 2: BRAID

As I have mentioned previously, pulling your hair to one side and placing in a loose braid will make it easier to sleep on and reduce matting from perspiration.

TIP 3: THE BACK-UP

As discussed above, what always worked best for me was to have two identical wigs; one that was specifically for sleeping over when having intimacy and the other to keep fresh for every day uses.

I would make love and then go to the ladies room and change into my thrasher wig to sleep in. Since the lights were out, he never noticed the difference in wigs; if anything, he just thought if it were messy it was a result of our romping! Then, I'd get up at least twenty minutes before he did, go to the bathroom, and change out of my thrasher wig and back into my gorgeous piece he had seen me in last, to avoid any notice or possible change in my hair.

I know you're probably thinking; that's an interesting move or what a pain to have to go through all that. But the truth is, this little move takes only seconds and has never failed me.

Men have always been oblivious to this, as they've been too caught up in the moment (thank God). I adore men, however I have found most to be a bit more linear than women and do better when concentrating on one thing at a time. Especially when it comes to intimacy and sex. Most of the time your partner will be so caught up in you, that he wouldn't (and shouldn't), pay enough attention to your hair to notice.

Here we go:

To pull this off successfully you need that extra thrasher wig, identical to the one you are wearing, along with The ResQ Bag™. My lovers never found out until I decided to tell them. (And it's far better than the alternative – having to expose my secret before I was ready to.) Get close – begin your fondling – then cutely and nonchalantly, excuse yourself to the ladies room saying you just need a minute. Make sure the door is closed, remove your current wig and turn it inside out; immediately place it in a ResQ Bag™ or if you don't have one, you can place it in a large zip lock baggie. Leave a small amount of air in the baggie as that will keep the wig fluffy. If you take air out of the bag, the wig will flatten out.

Sex, Wigs and Whispers

When we're nervous we can forget the most important things and you want to keep your discretion; so place the wig in the **bottom** of your bag. I would go to the extreme of wrapping a scarf around the zip lock baggie. Remember the key is keeping your secret regardless of how nervous and excited you may be – especially if that's your intention.

Attach one side of the wig tape to the front and each side of temples and nape; do this prior to placing it in the ResQ Bag™ or baggie. To do this correctly 'in a rush' be sure to remove <u>only one side</u> of the tape before placing it on each tape tab; this is so the part facing up is covered with the wig tape, thus preventing it from catching on to the other hair. You'll remove the remaining cover when you're ready to put the wig on. This technique will help when you are in a hurry to get back in that room!

Note: To help keep your secret, be sure to hide the discarded wig tape papers either in your bag or if you must – then make sure to wrap it tightly in tissue a few times in a ball and place it on the bottom of partner's waste basket. One of my biggest mistakes was when I threw them in the toilet, causing it to overflow! (I told him "they were from my makeup." Luckily he bought it... Don't ask – talk about ruining the mood!)

AFFIRMATION

I am unafraid to take on any challenge because I know now that I have the tools to get me through any situation that arises. I am fully in control and prepared to enjoy intimacy and sex without fear.

Hello, Fellatio!

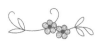

"Women complain about premenstrual syndrome, but I think of it as the only time of the month that I can be myself... hysterical."

Roseanne Barr

Due to the positioning, this can be an interesting, super fun challenge. Since I had to ask my honey to actually volunteer *his* body part, writing this chapter turned into a hysterical session, allowing me to document all my positions. Yes ladies, there I was on my knees just for you and there he stood 'loud and proud,' while I did my best to reenact this sexual encounter for you. Don't ask what transpired to keep him in the 'necessary state of readiness' — hilarious! Suffice to say, we were creative…

I had my pad and paper next to me, as I patiently wrote down all the positions of the moment until he said,

"Come on already, Honey! I don't think I can do this much longer."

To which I quickly looked up and replied — "Think about baseball!"

Okay Ladies, here we go…

TIP 1: ON YOUR KNEES:

If on your knees, likely he has placed his hand on your hair; take one of your free hands and place it on his penis; as he continues to touch your hair, calmly take his hand off your head and place it on top of your hand, now on his penis.

You are now both masturbating your man. As you lean in to please him orally, you can calmly move his hand away from yours while his brain is centering on the anticipation of your forthcoming Fellatio.

If your man goes for your hair again, don't jolt! Calmly and in a soft sexy way, move your hand under his, so your hand in now on your hair, placing you in control.

Sex, Wigs and Whispers

While working on his penis, take your thumb and slowly rub the outside of his hand or under his palm. At times. I found this move to be like rubbing my tummy and patting my head at the same time, but with a little practice it quickly became an easy move for me to refer to. You can use this move while lying down as well.

TIP 2: LYING DOWN:

If lying down: You can use a different approach by removing his hands off your hair and gently but firmly at the same time placing them by his side, then begin to stroke his lower tummy, increasing his anticipation of your forthcoming Fellatio, thereby getting his attention back on to him and his body. Compliment him, tell him how handsome he is, how perfect he is, whatever your man likes to hear. Then, move onto giving him pleasure.

Practice makes perfect ladies and I promise they'll forget about your hair or lack of it!

AFFIRMATION

I can be in control of my every move during sex without fear about my wig. I can have fun, move the way I want, and excite my partner freely with an open heart.

On the Tip of His Tongue

"Decide whether or not the goal is worth the risk involved. If it is, stop worrying."

Amelia Earhart

How to hide your wig when your partner is looking 'up' at you.

If you're lying on your back and your partner is about to give you oral sex, just before you get lost in the moment or hopefully many moments – MAKE SURE the edge of your wig doesn't show in the front and the sides.

This is also true for a foot massage or anything else that finds you lying on your back with your lover looking up at you and you looking down at him.

TIP:

Take a small piece of tape – and cut it 1/8" wide by 1" in length and line it up to place it on the wig, just a smidgen beyond the edge of the frontal hairline of the wig. Press the tape down, attaching it to the base, and continue to pull down the remainder of the wig so that the nape is even with yours. This will help secure the front of the hair and prevent it from lifting during the heat of the moment.

Note: I did this only when needed (and if the lights are on) as doing this too often can take hair out of your piece. You want to be careful when removing the hair from the tape with a comb or brush to prevent loss of hair. It is for this reason that I use this tip sparingly.

If your hair falls in your face, take a little saliva and move your hair back away from your face.

I always have my stylists make light sideburns on the side of my wig and cut little baby hair along the frontal hairline, which will hide the edge of the wig (See Styling section).

Sex, Wigs and Whispers

As you're looking down at your lover, make sure you keep your chin down just a bit so he ends up looking at the top of your bangs, instead of underneath them. This always works great, however, it's difficult to hold this position, so use it wisely.

AFFIRMATION

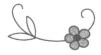

I am ready to enjoy sex and intimacy freely.
I'm ready to have fun!
I'm ready to try new things, new processes and new techniques, knowing that I am always Divinely protected and guided.

Sex, Wigs and Whispers

Shower Me with Your Love

HOW TO SHOWER WITH YOUR LOVER

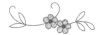

"The way to get started is to quit talking and begin doing."

Walt Disney

As we've discussed, with all wig intimacy the secret here is to get all the attention off of you, and on to him. If your partner reaches over to touch your hair, take his hand and put it somewhere else. Hold his hand to your face, place it on your heart, hold it to your lips or... put it where the sun don't shine! Anywhere but your head, hair, or the back of your neck.

Most of the time, showering with your boyfriend is not something that is planned days ahead. It's something that is born out of the heat of passion. That's why it's important to have the tools you need at your fingertips so you can relax and enjoy the moment.

Showering together is an extraordinary way to enhance a passionate experience with your lover. But for a wig wearer, this can be challenging and frightening. The secret to showering with your partner is actually a lot easier than you think.

It will depend on three things:

1) The type of wig you are wearing.

2) A good adhesive or wig clips to keep your piece adhered to your head and a wig that will hold up in water.

3) 'Acting' as if all is normal. *WHAT, you say!?*

As mentioned throughout this book, others pick up on your vibe (energy) first. Know that most people are really unaware of wigs and the entire process and most of the time would never notice anything is different about you unless <u>*you*</u> start to act differently.

Just because you're wearing a wig doesn't mean you can't enjoy warm sexy moments. During intimacy, don't be afraid to go under the water *together* – your hair will be fine.

Sex, Wigs and Whispers

Go for it, have a fabulous time and don't worry. Just follow these suggestions and stay calm. You'll be fine.

TIP 1:

*Certain wigs can handle water better than others. The CreatedHair.Com Heat Resistant Hair fiber **likes** water. The CyberHair® wigs we offer are made of a high spun nylon and has built in buoyancy, so it doesn't drag when it gets wet like human hair has a tendency to do. When you swim in our collection of Active Wigs it has a similar feel to hair that is floating away from you; it's that light. That's why we say, "It's like wearing air."*

Regular synthetic wigs can handle getting wet. It's just the cap base that can become an issue. If you are wearing an open wefted piece, be careful as the spaces in between each weft separate more easily, thus exposing the wig cap. Hand-tied pieces and closed wefted caps work better when wet. If you have a bit of your own hair, this is not as much of an issue as it is for those with no hair. However, the weft can still show, so be careful and try your particular wig out first before showering. This way, you are well-prepared and at ease, making the experience more comfortable for you.

Here are two ways to shower:

1) *Those who want to get their hair wet.*

2) *Those who do not want to get their hair wet.*

TIP 2: FOR THOSE WHO WANT TO GET THEIR HAIR WET, FOLLOW THESE INSTRUCTIONS.

When you get into the shower, step in and try to wash parts of your body first, easing into it, without putting your head all the way under the water yet.

When you're ready to place your hair under the water, do not scrub it or it will tangle. Just like the "Wig Maintenance" chapter, do not rinse by flopping your head over, as that will also cause tangling. Always make sure the water is going in the same direction as your hair.

If you decide to wash your hair just make sure to pour a little shampoo in your hands and stroke it through the wig with your fingers. Once again, Do Not Scrub or you will tangle the hair in your piece. Rinse – let the water wash the shampoo off in the correct direction as mentioned above. Repeat with conditioner. Work the suds through your hair with your fingers.

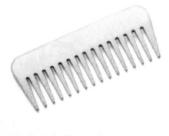

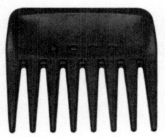

You can also take a wide tooth comb and slowly work the conditioner through the hair. Rinse as instructed. Careful not to place conditioner on the root of the hair at the crown or top of wig, as it has a tendency to loosen the knots, resulting in loss of hair.

Sex, Wigs and Whispers

TIP 3: FOR THOSE WHO DO NOT WANT TO GET THEIR HAIR WET, FOLLOW THESE INSTRUCTIONS.

As you step into the shower place your body – hips first and then the rest of your body, facing forward, rinsing off the front of you first... You can rinse off without letting the water touch your hair by arching your back. If it does get wet don't panic – it will dry.

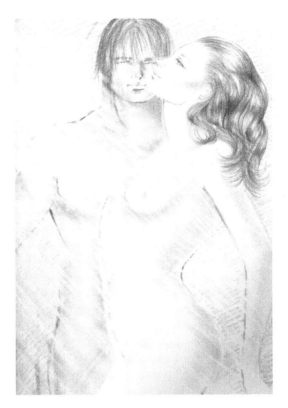

If you're wearing synthetic hair it will dry pretty quickly – the longer the hair, the longer the dry-time. Human hair will take longer to dry unless it's very short. I know we are all used to taking our wet hair, wrapping it in a towel, followed by rubbing it dry in a brisk fashion. You can still wrap your hair in a towel if you prefer. However, since this is non-breathing hair that easily tangles, try not to rub so hard.

Shower Me With Your Love

Remember, you're trying to be inconspicuous, so don't change how you would normally dry your hair; just do so lightly and a bit more carefully.

It is for these reasons that I suggest Heat Resistant hair because it's great for sports, dancing and anything to do with water.

Most importantly, try to stay in the moment, be present with your lover, and not be caught up in "your hair;" you will lose out on this great moment with your man. Instead, be caught up in him, and he will not only get more excited, but be caught up in you, and the two of you will embrace the experience, thereby creating a stronger connection.

AFFIRMATION

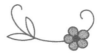

I am finally at ease with this entire wig shower process and capable of handling it with absolute grace. I am able to enjoy stepping into the shower and concentrating only on my lover's lips.

Sex, Wigs and Whispers

Beach Love

*"Life is 10% of what happens to me and
90% of how I react to it."*

John Maxwell

$S$and and the beach have long been linked with romance and love. It's also a wonderful haven for ants and little 'buggers.'

TIP:

If you are on the sand, even on a towel or a blanket, be sure that when you get up you shake your hair out immediately, then 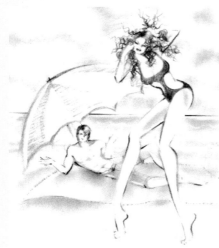 *take a brush and gently comb through your hair. If you see a bug or two, don't do what I have done in the past; like jump and scream while pulling on my hair to get the bugs out. (I hate bugs!) All that does is make you look like a weird wimp, made worse when your wig falls off. This one I know from experience!*

If you're wearing alternative hair, spraying a 'little" (a bit more than a mist) of hair spray on the piece will keep the hair in place. Wrapping your hair in a bun or ponytail also helps diminish those buggers access into your hair.

These tips work anytime you're at the beach and in the sand.

AFFIRMATION

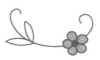

I will live the life I want now.
I wait for nothing and no one to move my life forward.

Sex, Wigs and Whispers

Assume The Position

"If you're going to do something tonight that you'll be sorry for in the morning, sleep late."

Henny Youngman

Before beginning this experience, if you are really uncomfortable with anyone handling your hair, remember we've discussed what you can say;

"Listen, I got a hair treatment and my head is a bit sensitive, so I'd appreciate it if you wouldn't touch my head or my hair tonight. (Coyly...) You can touch anything else... just not my hair."

This is where that smile I mentioned earlier really comes in handy!

One of the most difficult moments for a woman wearing a wig is when you're lying down on your back, thereby squashing wig hair against the pillow. You have no mirror to make sure the wig is still on straight and no one to tell you that your hair is flying in a hundred different directions! Wigs, if not made in a thin light base, can get hot and itchy, and create perspiration, which causes the hair to mat and tangle. If you're wearing a synthetic piece, by the time you arise, your hair is standing at attention, just like your man was!

The pitfalls of being on your back:

- Wig gets matted and tangled
- Moving your head around may show wig

So how do you deal with this?

TIP 1: WIG GETS MATTED AND TANGLED

As I mention in the chapter Your Bed or Mine, invest in a satin pillowcase; it will lessen the amount of static. Satin sheets are romantic too, so it's easy to get away with. If you're not in your own surroundings and your partner doesn't take well to our suggestion of "loving satin sheets," then turn your wig upside down, and while holding the nape, carefully brush out your wig from the inside of the nape down as soon as possible.

Sex, Wigs and Whispers

TIP 2: MOVING YOUR HEAD AROUND

Always carry a few bobby pins for added security. If you're wearing tape and feeling a bit concerned, discreetly tape each one and hold down for a second to further secure it's adhering to your scalp. This may help calm whatever anxiety you have. If by chance you have forgotten your tape, some types of tape can be reactivated by dabbing a little bit of 99% alcohol on the tape with a q-tip. In those times when I have forgotten my tape – I've even used packing tape by turning it inside out, and making it a completed circle, so the sticky part can attach to both the wig base and my head.

Putting your hair in a quick braid will help keep the hair in place. Pulling a little hair from the side will add a more realistic look and hide the edge of the wig, thus increasing your comfort level. You can lure him into helping you with the braiding process, making it quite a sensual experience for you both.

Put your hair on one side. Make sure your head is on the pillow and then subtly and sensually, calmly start to braid your hair as he stares lustfully into your eyes. If he starts to pull his hand through your hair, take your hands and place them immediately on the outside of his hands; it can get very sensual by squeezing his hands tightly. Slowly take his hands off your hair – again – and place them 'elsewhere.'

TIP 3:

Remember, quick moves can confuse a person and certainly break the mood and then that 'weird dance' begins. So remember that you are always in control and can take as much time you as want!

So go ahead girls, enjoy.

Assume the Position

AFFIRMATION

*All I need is a little preparation, knowledge and trust,
and I can successfully handle any intimate moment.*

Pedi Time

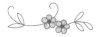

You are now at a crossroads.
This is your opportunity to make
the most important decision
you will ever make.
Forget your past.
Who are you now?

Who have you decided you really are now?
Don't think about who you have been.
Who are you now?
Who have you decided to become?
Make this decision consciously.
Make it carefully.
Make it powerfully.

Tony Robbins

How to give your man a pedicure while you're looking down at his feet without worrying about him focusing on the top or crown of your wig.

This is for doing anything when someone is looking down at your head.

How do you proceed?

TIP:

This tip is all about angles – the angle at which you place him and the angle in which you place yourself. It will be far better for him to be elevated in front of you and you look up towards him, rather than you facing down at him. I usually place him on the edge of the bed and sit on a stool a bit lower or I place him on the couch and myself on the lower ottoman. This way, you prevent him from being able to see up – into your frontal hairline.

AFFIRMATION

Today I take on a new perspective.
Today I choose to take the first step into
who I want to become and how I want to live.
I do this consciously and with absolute focus on
only the positive result I am creating for myself.

Ruff Ruff

*"Goals are the fuel
in the furnace of achievement."*

Brian Tracy, Eat that Frog

WHEN YOUR LOVER IS BEHIND YOU – pulling on your hair in the heat of passion.

This is a highly desirable position, done with frequency and can be very physical. It involves holding and even pulling the hair, which can definitely be challenging; but not impossible… it just takes some sexy maneuvering.

Once again, this ever repeating tip rings true here: the secret for all wig intimacy is that every time your partner goes to reach for your hair – keep placing the attention back onto him and off your hair.

I have found that in the beginning of my hair loss journey, as my guy would go to grab my hair I would immediately tense up, become rigid and/or my stomach would be in a knot. Then I learned that there were easier and fun ways to handle the situation. For both of us!

TIP 1: LEAD THE WAY:

Since many women (and men) love this position, it's important to learn how to participate and enjoy as you always have! These are a few diversions during lovemaking as you find his hands in your hair;

"Oooh not my hair babe, but I'd LUV it on my hips!

"Go ahead, pull my hips deeper into you."

"Take my Lips, babe"

"'Pull me into you – let me feel you!"

"Grab my ass! (That should get him off your hair!)

Sex, Wigs and Whispers

Be creative and imaginative. It will cause your lover to pull you into him, rather than pull onto your hair; and that just feels better for everybody!

TIP 2: GO FOR THE SHOULDERS:

"Oh baby, pulling my hair doesn't do it for me. Grab my shoulders – I love it when you do that. You feel so strong."

TIP 3: GET HIM HOT. TALK YOUR WARMEST, MOST SENSUAL, SEXIEST TALK.

He'll respond to anything when he's lit up!

If all this is too awkward for you then use the following if this feels comfortable for you (Or tell your partner something along the lines of...):

Ohh honey, I had a color treatment recently and my hair is soo sensitive so please be kind to "her" – anything below the shoulders is a go! (With a smile of course)

AFFIRMATION

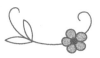

*I am totally capable of enjoying the moment.
I am at ease and in control of every decision I make.
I approach sex in an entirely different and positive way now.
I have the means to control my man
and where he puts his hands with absolute ease.*

Ruff Ruff

Sex, Wigs and Whispers

Shake Your Booty

"Children's talent to endure stems from their ignorance of alternatives."

Maya Angelou

It's time to go dancing...

Dancing is dancing and if done with abandon, the only way I know how to do it, your precious 'little lady' should be downright wet! When this happens, do the following...

TIP:

Excuse yourself for a moment to the nearest ladies room. Grab a paper towel or tissue and dampen slightly. For discretionary purposes, take a private stall. Then, completely remove the piece, which will allow you to wipe your head and neck area fully with the dampened towel. If you're wearing 2-sided wig tape, take a moment to pat your head dry and change the wig tape on your piece before placing it back on your head.

If caught without a mirror, remember when putting on a wig the temples need to rest evenly on both sides. So place the wig lightly on your head, close your eyes and concentrate on how both temples feel. Are they even? Is one higher than the other? If so, just give a little tug and straighten it out. Place the front of the wig at your hairline and bring down the back of the wig to where it's most comfortable on the nape.

If you find it too difficult to do this without a mirror, no worries. Place the wig on your head close to what you feel is the correct position and wait until where you can locate a mirror to position the piece correctly. Then with the wig in position, either press down on the wig tape or clips thereby securing it.

I have secured my wig alongside five other girls at the mirror, putting on their makeup and not one of them caught on. I just did what I had to do in a relaxed, 'very nonchalant fashion' and no one caught on. I love it!

Sex, Wigs and Whispers

Regardless of the length of time your date has waiting been for you while you located the mirror in the bathroom, take the time you need and honor yourself. That's what any secure woman would do, with or without hair.

You may want to think about making a small investment for a portable wig bag that can carry all those little things you may need so you have those tools for any spontaneous situation. It is for this reason that I created **The ResQ Bag**™.

If you don't want to carry all your accessories for use "later that evening," make sure to carry extra tape, 1 or 2 small individually wrapped scalp towelettes which you can purchase from CreatedHair.com or you pick up a box of witch hazel pads that will work just fine, and a needle and thread in case your wig clip comes loose. As we've discussed, "Preparation" is key to wig success.

Now go rock!

AFFIRMATION

I always take positive action in the face of fear.
I never stand down.

PART
7

Styling

Maintenance

How to Wash Your Wig

Feel free to follow along on YouTube:

PART 1: http://www.youtube.com/watch?v=Aykh52pUnyY

PART 2: http://www.youtube.com/watch?v=kFA5fYJ_P4Y

Remember: The Water Wig™, as well as regular synthetic pieces on the market, are easier to work with as they react more easily than human hairpieces which need more styling and care. However have no fear, once you understand how they work you'll have this down in no time!

To achieve the most success you'll need the following:

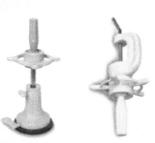

A Wig Clamp which holds the wig in place for styling.

I am often asked, *"How often do I need to wash it?"*

Depending on how much you wear the piece and your level of perspiration, I always say, *"You'll always know when the piece needs to be refreshed."* When 'she' begins to stop moving freely, looks and/or feels greasy, or has an unattractive fragrance, is when she needs a relaxing bath!

Do not use regular shampoo or hairspray on your piece, as it may contain ingredients like alcohol, which will dry out the hair. If wearing synthetic hair – it's best to only use products designed for synthetic hair wigs and hair pieces. The same goes for human hair. Although CreatedHair.com offers synthetic and human hair maintenance products with easy directions that will help extend the shelf life of your "investment", there are a few wig companies that will also make products to service both synthetic and human hair.

John Paul Mitchell, WEN, BedHead, Pantene and It's a Ten all work well. If interested inquire at: Book@CreatedHair.com for any maintenance products you may desire and we'll walk you through the process.

Optional Styling Gel or Hair Spray can be used for finishing as long as they don't contain alcohol.

– OKAY HERE WE GO –

Step 1. Pin

Pin your piece onto your wig head using <u>very</u> <u>small</u> pins. You can also use pins 1 1/2"- 2" in length. To hold the wig in place, you can use T-Pins as pictured below or purchase ones with the small balls at the end.

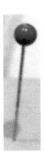 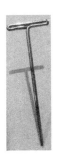 Place 1 pin at each side of sideburn area, 1 pins at right and left side of nape, and one pin in frontal hairline. If you have a lace front piece, I suggest you **do not place any pins on any part of the lace** as it will tear. If at all possible, try to place pins behind the lace where base material begins.

Step 2. Detangle

Comb hair first to remove tangles. "It's A Ten" De-tangler is a terrific product to use both on human hair and synthetic hair. There are others as well. If wearing synthetic, a wide tooth comb is suggested to use to help prevent and remove tangles.

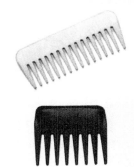

Step 3: Basin

Fill basin with lukewarm or cold water.

Step 4: Shampoo

There are two techniques you can use for applying shampoo and/or conditioner:

a) Place a small amount of shampoo on your hands and run it through the strands of the hair.

b) Fill a basin or bowl with warm water and add a tablespoon of shampoo to the water.

    After placing the piece in water, move it from left to right in an easy flow through motion. You can dunk the piece straight up and down. **Warning: Never twirl the piece in any circular motion or it will tangle.**

Step 5. Rinse

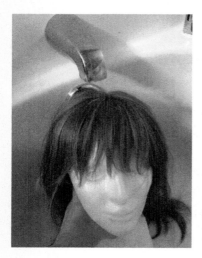

There are three techniques you can use to rinse.

1)   Hold wig head at the base directly under the faucet allowing the water to rinse the hair in one direction. (See pic at left)

2)   Turn wig inside out, re-attach piece to wig head, and follow directions above to rinse hair in one direction.

3) Rinse sink or basin and replace with fresh water. Place the piece in water, move it from left to right in an easy flow through motion following shampoo directions above.

Sex, Wigs and Whispers

Step 6. Condition

Warning: When applying a small amount of conditioner directly to the hair, avoid getting conditioner on the base or root as it tends to loosen the knots.

Leave on for a few minutes and rinse using the same technique employed for rinsing out the shampoo in #5.

Step 7. Drying the Piece

Place wet item on either a friction free absorbent towel (available at CreatedHair.com) or regular towel and blot gently on a hard surface.

Do not rub the wet hair or it will cause it to tangle. Avoid brushing the wet piece, but rather allow to air dry by placing over on a wig head in your <u>correct size</u> that will not stretch the base.

Alternative: Placing the piece on a wire or plastic wig stand fits any size wig and allows for easier ventilation and faster drying time.

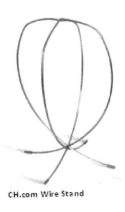

CH.com Wire Stand

Avoid using heat (especially on synthetic fiber). Only use a blow dryer w/ cool air or on low heat with caution. (Refer to Styling Chapter for instruction on using heat products).

Optional Styling Gel and Hair Spray can be used at any time. However please use sparingly whenever using these products to avoid having to wash the piece more often than needed.

To Create Height: Hang the wig to dry upside down. To do this, take a clip hanger and as if you are looking at the inside of the

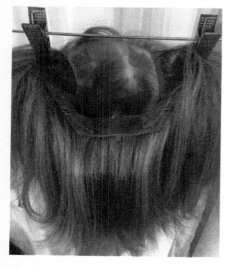

base, attach either end of the sideburns to the clip hanger. Hang until dry. After 'she' is dry, you'll have height and may even need to calm the style by patting 'her' down a bit!

If you want the 'stick up' look, just spray a little bit of strong hairspray or mousse on your hands, then rub your hands together and simply run your fingers through your hair. The hair will go in the direction you place it.

If you want to have the ends flip up, rub some mousse between your hands and run your fingers through your hair and then as you get to the ends, grab the ends, turn them up and let go. Basically, just guide the hair into the style you want.

To Create More Wave Naturally without using heat products: If you want the piece to be more wavy; after washing – pat it dry well and place the damp piece on a towel with the crown facing up and leave that way until fully dry. Brush though with your fingers or a wide-tooth comb.

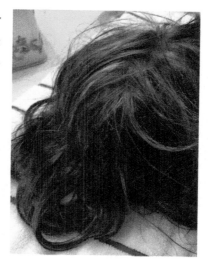

Hygiene – IMPORTANT – Always keep your scalp clean as it the closest thing to our brains!

ResQ Bag™ Towelettes work great; however, you an also use soap and water or toner on cotton ball.

Feel free to contact us at: Book@CreatedHair.com with any questions .

Enjoy!

Amy

Styling Section

"It is our choices that show what we truly are, far more than our abilities."

J.K. Rowling

BASE WIG CAPS

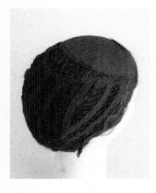

<u>Open Wefted Caps</u> – Open wefted caps have a natural skin top that resembles a scalp. From the crown to the nape, there are many wefts (rows of hair) sewn horizontally across from ear to ear. The area between each weft is open so the cap does not feel as tight on the head. When pinning a wig up, the open wefts allow the pins to go through the cap and be fastened to the hair growing from the head, which assures a firm hold. The open wefts also allow more ventilation to the scalp. I do not recommend this type of cap for women with no hair as you see through the wefts to the scalp if the wind blows. These work fine for those with short or longer hair. Great for patients with 2-3" of hair regrowth following the completion of their chemotherapy treatment.

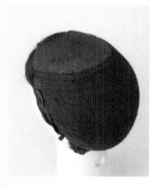

<u>Close Wefted Caps</u> – Closed wefted caps have a natural skin top that resembles a scalp. From the crown to the nape, there is a single piece of stretch material covering the wefts that are sewn horizontally across from ear to ear. This cap has a snugger fit and because the single piece of material is completely closed to the head, it prevents hair from the head from coming through. Due to the snug fit, many women wearing wigs for Alopecia or wigs for cancer prefer the closed wefted cap.

Sex, Wigs and Whispers

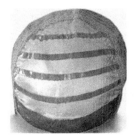

Hand-Tied and Close Wefted Caps can also include small strips of silicone that help the cap adhere to the scalp. However, silicone placed in a cap works best with no hair. Depending on fit, this usually will remove the need for tape.

INVERSION

Inversion is when hair seeps back though the inside of the cap. It can be a problem with synthetic and human hair pieces.

The most common reason for this is caused by not using a wig head during washing. Using a properly-sized foam or canvas wig head will prevent the water from pushing the hairs back through the base.

In a wefted piece (a long string of hair fiber attached to a piece of material that is doubled over and sewn closely together), I have found that if you turn the wig upside down and brush it from the base to the end of the hair, it will many times pull some of the hair back out through the wig to the other side. With hand-tied pieces some of the hair can go back in, just not as easily. Since all hand-tied pieces are more delicate and susceptible to inversion, they require a bit more attention during maintenance and must always be washed while pinned on a wig head.

PROPERLY BRUSHING YOUR WIG

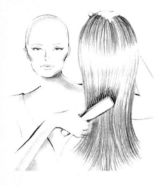

When brushing hair: Start from the bottom and work your way up to the crown. Then, after working your way to the crown do complete strokes from the top of the head down to the end. However, as I've mentioned, never pull on the hair as it will cause frizz and breakage.

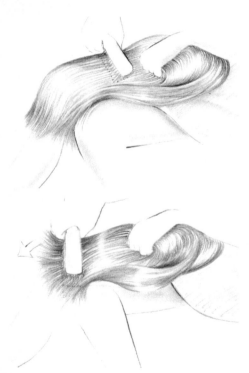

Sometimes placing the wig on your thigh and brushing the hair against your leg, will put less strain on the hair and allow you to see the knots more clearly, making it a safer, easier process.

If you encounter a knot, spray the hair with a 'little' "It's a Ten" De-Tangler or Argan oil. Now hold the area of hair in question and with the end of a rat-tail comb, try to gently, lovingly work through the knot. Be careful not to pull on the hair or you will stretch or break the hair fiber. Also, pulling on the hair fiber can cause it to frizz and expand. Wide-tooth combs are great for reducing tangles as well.

Sex, Wigs and Whispers

Reminders:

- Always use a clean comb and keep it in a clean storage after.

- Clean your combs every week. Don't forget to soak them in a mug with a mixture of warm water and shampoo. Vinegar mixed with lemon are good cleaning agents too.

- Use combs before and after shower. Don't use brushes.

- Go for combs with soft edges to avoid hurting your scalp

- Choose quality over quantity. Buy combs that are strong, avoid those that are breakable or can easily bend.

- Pick the right comb according to your hair type and texture.

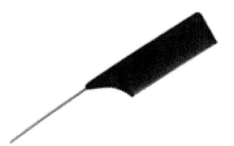

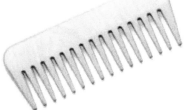

RAT-TAIL: A STANDARD RAT-TAIL COMB MEASURES FROM 8 TO 10 INCHES IN LENGTH. IT IS KNOWN FOR BEING ACCURATE IN SECTIONING THE HAIR HENCE, THE COMB WAS DESIGNED WITH VERY FINE AND CLOSELY POSITIONED TEETH WHILE THE POINTED END'S LIKE THAT OF A STRAIGHTENED RAT'S TAIL, INTENDED FOR PULLING SECTIONS OF HAIR. THIS TOOL IS ALSO ESSENTIAL FOR PUTTING HAIR EXTENSIONS AND PERFORMING CHEMICAL TREATMENTS.

WIDE-TOOTH COMB

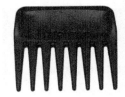

BABY HAIR

Baby hair is what we refer to as the small amount of hair mainly around the frontal hairline and some around the sides and nape. The other thing it does is camouflage the front edge of the wig. This adds a natural look to any wig, giving the impression of this being your own baby hair coming from your scalp. The other thing it does is to camouflage the front edge of the base of the wig.

It's best to have your hairstylist to do this. However if you want 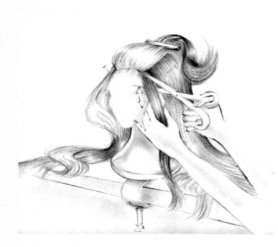 to try this yourself do the following: First pin your wig firmly into place onto a foam or canvas wig head at the front, sides and nape. From the front edge of the cap go back 1/10" inch. Take a comb and part the hair going across horizontally. You should not be holding a lot of hair. Since the hair has a habit of sticking out after working on in it in this fashion, you want to make sure the hair is directed downward. Depending on the look you care to attain, take a curling or straightening iron and run through the area of hair you just worked on.

Take a small amount of hair about 1/8 of inch from this bunch you just measured.

Now hold and pull the small amount of hair straight down. Open a pair of well sharpened scissors and run the inner edge of the scissors in an upward motion against the hair.

Note: Be careful to leave a little room and not to close the scissors completely or you'll cut into the hair too deeply.

This is referred to as shredding. The secret is to do this with a small amount of hair to create the real baby effect.

SIDEBURN BABY HAIR

Repeat and do the same for the sideburns.

NAPE HAIR

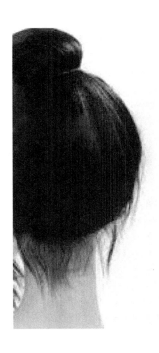

This is a terrific way to wear a pony tail and have it look like it's growing right out of your head! My young ballerinas love this technique as it creates such a natural look.

For this it's best to have a stylist do it for you while your wig is on your head. If no stylist is available, pin your piece to a wig head and follow these directions carefully.

The secret to achieving this natural look is to cut the last "ventilation" of hair (the last row of hair – very thin section) at the bottom of the nape. Part going across horizontally, once again, shred.

DEALING WITH FRIZZ

Frizz is most common with synthetic hair but matting and frizz can happen with human hair as well. So if you're going to be part of this wig wearing world, you better learn how to live within in it or you will forever be frustrated, not at peace or look your optimum best. And isn't living peacefully and joyfully while in this process our ultimate goal?

There are two good ways to get rid of Lady Frizz:

STEAM

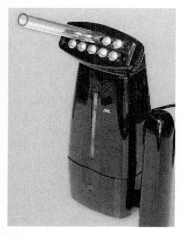

To do this you'll need a small travel steamer – preferably a steamer with a directional pipe.

Turn your wig inside out and pin it to a foam wig head as described on page 269.

Place small T-Pins at the sideburns, top and both sides of the nape. Make sure not to stretch the piece to fit the wig head. If the wig is too small, either purchase a small sized wig head or pin the wig without meeting all the usual edges of the foam wig head – resting loosely on the wig head, but again, still pinned down.

If the wig doesn't straighten all the way down, don't worry. For this process you just to make sure the back of the wig is straight and pinned down to cleanly get to the nape area.

Starting with the nape area, pin up a good portion of back of the hair on top with bobby pins or a clip. Take a small amount of the hair underneath the nape area and comb it going downward.

Warning: Keep in mind, hair that is not attached to the head lacks natural oils, so you must be careful with using heat products too often on your piece as it will dry your piece out and eventually ruin it. As with any heating tool you want to be careful not to leave it on the hair too long or hold too close on the hair or you'll burn it.

As you comb the hair downward, follow with the steamer holding it 6 inches above hair as you simultaneously brush the section again. Do this quickly so as not to burn it. The secret is after you have steamed the area of hair, you must let it cool in place for a 1-2 minutes; blowing on the piece after you have steamed it helps to quickly cool and set the fiber. You can pin it up and move on to the next small section. After your steaming is completed, take down all the hair and use your hand to work through the hair or softly brush through it.

USING A STRAIGHTENING IRON

For human hair you're safe with 350°. Some use 400° to 450°, but with any heat system you must be quick with your strokes when moving through the hair.

Synthetic hair should be 250° to be safe.

With any system, it is best to take a small amount of the hair and comb it going downward.

Warning: As with any heating tool you want to be careful not to leave it on the hair too long or hold too close on the hair or you'll burn it.

Use the straightening iron as we did with the steamer, by working with a small amount of hair, section by section in this process. Take a small section and lightly spritz it with water 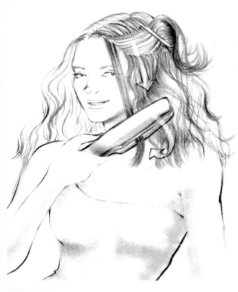 (Distilled water works well). I also like to use Aquage Working Spray. My stylist likes to use a light bit of hair spray on the area ('light' being the operative word here) and it works great; however, I find it gets sticky when I do it so I prefer to use water or the working spray.

Take a small section and place the hair in between the straightener − best to do towards the front or tip of the straightener as that usually grabs the most hair. Run down to the end of the hair no longer than 5 seconds. For a nice bend, you can turn the iron under at the end.

The secret is after you have straightened the area of hair, you must let it cool in place. You can pin it up or to the side away from the remaining hair and move on to the next small section. This adds curl back into your piece.

To use a curling iron, simply wrap a small amount of hair around the iron for 5-6 seconds and slowly loosen the grip leaving the curl in place. Blow on it to cool, then place the hair into pin curls, and put it to the side. This will help hold the curl. Often, "FRIZZY hair" is caused by using a flat or curling iron on hair that is still damp. This is why I stress to "lightly spritz a mist" when you applying water or any working spray. Since

Sex, Wigs and Whispers

heat styling breaks down the hair's hydrogen bonds, applying concentrated heat from a curling or straightening iron can be very damaging. It's optimum to wait until your hair is dry, or blow dry your hair on a low setting to speed the process along, before using an iron. Otherwise, you may cause irreversible damage to your strands.

Choosing the temperature of your heat styling tool should be according to the thickness and texture of your hair. If you have very thick or curly hair, you may find you need a higher heat setting to achieve the look you want. If your hair is thin or fine, then using a lower heat setting is suggested because a higher heat setting can burn hair. When deciding on how to style it, I suggest going with the natural texture of your hair. Begin with a lower heat setting and work your way up the temperature scale if you find you need it.

You don't need to spend a fortune and buy the most expensive tools on the market, but you should adhere to a few basic requirements when selecting your heat tools:

With flat irons and straighteners, look for products that offer different temperature controls and have high quality plates. Current technologies have helped straightening irons become less damaging, so if your flat iron is several years old, consider upgrading to a newer model. I prefer ionic flat irons, as they produce negative ions, which balance hair to eliminate static and frizz.

Most hair straighteners have plates made of ceramic, titanium, tourmaline or a combination of two. All of these materials produce negative ions when heated, which help to smooth, straighten and seal the cuticle of hair strands. However, each type is ideal for a different type of hair. Ceramic hair straighteners maintain high temperatures and even heat distribution, which results in shiny and frizz-free locks with minimal damage. Solid ceramic plates are more expensive than ceramic-coated plates, but they are not as prone to chipping or damaging hair. Ceramic flat irons are ideal for most hair types, ranging from thin to thick tresses.

Titanium plates also boast consistent heat and high temperatures. However, they boast higher ionic output than ceramic plates. A titanium hair iron is best suited for thick, undamaged and coarse hair that is difficult to straighten. If you have fine hair, you should only use this type of flat iron on the lowest temperature setting.

Unlike ceramic and titanium, tourmaline is not a standalone material; rather, it is a semi-precious stone that is crushed up and typically infused into ceramic or titanium plates. Plates infused with tourmaline are ideal for coarse hair because they reduce friction as you straighten your hair, resulting in ultra sleek locks.

The most basic and cheapest of flat irons have metal plates. They can flatten unruly tresses but are more likely to cause hair damage. Metal plates can have inconsistent temperatures across the surface, which can cause hot spots and, subsequently, damage to your hair. They also are not as smooth as ceramic or titanium plates and can cause friction as you pull your hair between the two plates. As you can see, there are many types of curling irons available; pick yours based on the size and shape of the curl you desire. For smaller, tighter curls use a smaller barrel. A larger barrel will create loose waves. Both looks are really popular and loose waves rock!

Blow dryers that have a nozzle attachment will distribute heat more evenly. For curly hair you may also want to invest in a diffuser head for your blow dryer to spread the heat. If you can afford it, salon-quality hair dryers, i.e. ionic or tourmaline dryers, typically have more powerful air flow than lower-quality blow dryers.

Caruso Ionic Steam Rollers are a wonderful way to implement curl without causing damage to the hair fiber. The key to using

Sex, Wigs and Whispers

them without getting the mark caused by the closing clip is to take the steam curler, wrap the desired small section of hair, and place a T-pin through the curler directly into the foam wig head.

Protecting your hair before styling

It's critical to protect your beautiful hair before applying heat. There are many hair care products designed for use with heat styling tools. Products you can spray on that contain silicone can act as a protective coating for your hair. The secret is distributing a 'small layer' of this silicone and not a heavy coating. **Warning**: Using standard products on "created hair" can cause serious damage, as you'll burn the styling products along with your hair! Make sure any product you apply before heat styling is specifically formulated for the type of hair you are working with.

Argan Oil, commonly referred to as "liquid gold", is a plant oil produced from the kernels of the argan tree (Argania spinosa L.) that is endemic to Morocco.

It delivers instant shine and helps to seal split ends and deliver intense moisture to each layer of the hair strand for long-lasting rejuvenation. Argan Oil naturally penetrates the hair to help moisturize each layer of the hair strand for long-term hair repair so your hair actually looks and feels healthier, silkier, and extraordinarily shiny.

To be safe, it's best to start out conservative when using oils on your hair. In your hands, mix a small amount (1 Teaspoon) of argon oil with a couple of pumps of hair spray and rub your hands together. Lightly run your hand throughout your hair. If you feel you didn't cover enough strands put a touch more on.

But be careful not to saturate the hair. This also helps to hold a curl.

Air dry when possible.

It's fab to go natural once in a while! It's good to give your hair a break from heat styling every once in a while. I suggest using a texturizing spray or mousse when you air-dry your hair, as these will add a little shape and volume to your style. If you have long or thick hair and hate leaving the house with wet hair, try washing it the night before and let it air dry naturally. Your hair will thank you!

STRETCHING THE WIG

Have several 1 7]8"- 2 1/2" T- Pins and spray bottle filled with regular water. Filtered or distilled are best if available. If not, regular water will do.

1) Turn wig inside out and place on a wig head.

2) Begin at the front of the wig and secure a T-pin into base and onto wig head. If you're wearing a lace-front piece, be careful not to place any pin directly into the lace at the front or it may tear. I would first play it safe by moving to the right and left of the front area, which are the "temples" area. I would try to place the pin in the area where the lace ends and base begins.

3) Spray the wig with a little water while inside out so it's slightly damp. DO NOT SOAK.

4) Pull the wig straight down and work your fingers through the wig to the nape, pulling back as you go and then take the nape and securely pin the bottom of the nape in place.

5) Work your way around the wig; keep pinning on one side while stretching across and pinning the opposite side.

Once you are sure you have gotten all the stretch you can get out the base while being careful not to tear it, then spray around the edge of the base lightly with water. Place in a cool spot and let it sit for 2-3 days before carefully removing pins to avoid ripping base.

If needed, you can then repeat the process all over again and let it sit for another day or two before removing from wig head.

THINNING THE WIG WITHOUT SHEARS

REMOVING DENSITY SAFELY AND EVENLY FROM YOUR WIG

Products needed for this tip:

- Nair Hair Removal Lotion or Cream
- Major patience
- Focus and... a good toothpick!

Section off the area of hair you want thinned. Make sure you don't take too much hair at a time or you risk the Nair spreading on hair you don't want thinned and leaving you with a possible a bald spot.

I did that once when one day I decided to replicate my wax salon and Nair my pubic hair myself. I set out to create the perfect feminine "hello." I carefully placed the Nair in the perfect areas between my thighs and then began to wait – Oh – but then I got an important call, so I took a seat.

That's right I crossed my legs and proceeded to have a great gab when I suddenly realized I had been talking for almost 30 minutes… needless to say, I didn't end up with the design I had in mind! What started out as a Picasso was now an airplane strip! It grew back…

Obviously we needn't illustrate – LOL! Ok – back to work –

Comb through the section of the hair until smooth. If it tangles use a small amount of de-tangler or conditioning product on the section before applying Nair Hair Removal.

Do a small strand test first on the piece to get you used to using this process and seeing how the hair reacts. To do this, take the hair on top – place it aside and pin it, making sure it's away from the working area.

I prefer not to take the hair from the top of the crown but instead work from underneath the first layer.

Lightly dampen the small area you will be working on.

Pour Nair on a plate.

Dip the end of toothpick in the Nair - careful not to put too much on the toothpick.

Lightly place the toothpick with the Nair on only the root of the damp hair.

Now take your finger and lightly bring the Nair through the hair with your fingers. Don't press down on the area, or you'll end up with a bald spot. DO NOT COMB THROUGH YET OR YOU WILL HAVE NO CONTROL OVER THE AMOUNT OF LOSS OF YOUR HAIR.

Sex, Wigs and Whispers

Leave it on for 10 minutes. To test if it's ready – now, comb through the test strands to see how much hair had released. If no or little hair has released, leave on for 5 more minutes and re-test. You should not need to leave on longer than 20 minutes.

After you have tested the first strand – washed it out and brushed the hair out of the area, thus removing unwanted hair which should have released easily – you should be feeling more secure of the outcome you have received.

Carefully repeat, working your way around the wig while still continuing the work with the underneath layers.

Once you've covered a particular area, move on to make sure you don't end up with uneven symmetry in your piece. You want to end up with even density all around, having the finished look being less hair all over, giving it an overall lighter, more natural look.

If after blow drying you find that more hair removal is needed then carefully do so. As I said, this process takes patience. If you find that after you have finished working with the underneath of the piece, the crown and top is still too heavy, then VERY carefully remove one to three hairs at a time in different areas by applying a 'dot' of Nair to the areas using the tooth pick ONLY and not your fingers. As this is most obvious area you want to take your time.

IMPORTANT NOTES:

- Dip only the end of toothpick in the Nair – careful not to put too much on the toothpick.

- Place the Nair on only the root of the damp hair.

HOW TO EXTEND HER SHELF LIFE!

Ladies, we spend good money on our little ladies so let's make them last as long as we can!

Just Follow These 3 Easy Steps:

Storing

When storing your wig either place it on a foam wig head or wire wig stand, roll your wig neatly into a wig box, or store it safely in the ResQ Bag™.

To do this, place your wig on her "back" so the inside of the wig is facing you. Take the sides and fold them inward towards the center. Take the top/ bang area and roll down into the wig while tucking in the sides you go.

Alternative: ResQ Bag™

Take your wig in one hand and with your free hand twirl the wig in a soft circular motion. Take the bottom of the hair and softly roll into the cap of the wig to make an even ball. Place into inner Mini ResQ Bag™ with the cap of the wig facing upwards. Tuck loose hair gently inside cap. If storing Extensions into the inner Mini ResQ Bag™, continue laying the hair in a circle. Pull tab to tighten.

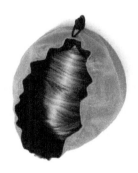

Box/Plastic bag

Place in a box preferably with a lid or a plastic bag. If using a bag make sure to leave some air in the bag or the wig will be flattened. Never store near heat.

Sex, Wigs and Whispers

Using a De-Tangler /Conditioner

"It's A Ten" Miracle spray is brilliant for releasing matting or tangles. Just take one small section at a time, spray a "little" on the area and then slowly comb through the hair with a wide tooth comb. Be careful to use sparingly, or the piece will look greasy.

Our little ladies take a bit of patience but it's worth it!

TAPE TABS

As not all wig bases will adhere to wig tape, Tape Tabs are made of small, extremely thin translucent pieces of Polyurethane material that are easily sewn into a wig cap for added security. You can purchase them from CreatedHair.com or some fabric stores. Tape Tabs are one of 12 complimentary essential accessories included in the ResQ Bag™.

Basically it's like sewing on a button.

Get clear nylon thread or a neutral color polyester thread if you're in the lighter shades, or darker thread if in the darker shades to blend in with your wig, as the thread can easily show through the base.

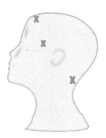
Sew the tape tabs with the shiny side facing toward you onto the wig where needed. Most women prefer 1 at the front hair line, 1 at the sides/temples and 2 at either side of the nape. If they come off just sew them back on or purchase some material for future use.

TWO-SIDED WIG TAPE

Yes ladies, for those of you who may be unaware, you no longer have to be concerned with your wig flying off or sliding to the left when you least expect it!

Wig tape needs a clean scalp to adhere to. It does not adhere to hair very well and you'll end up tearing your hair out. Not recommended.

Note: Some tape is stronger than others. When using stronger bonding tape or the CreatedHair Water Wig tape, do not try to peel off both sides of the tape and place on your finger first or it will curl up and be unusable. Since it's two sided, just peel off one side of the tape, place directly onto the cap, remove the other side of the tape, place on your head, and you're ready to go.

Best places are at the temples, right and left side of nape and frontal hair line.

If you have hair loss but good side burns and can afford to shave a teeny weeny bit in the very front of the side burn, frontal hairline and/or just below your natural nape hairline, then cut tape into very thin strips (1/8 of an inch) and place there to adhere and secure your piece.

For those of you with some hair or those of you who are not going to use your own bangs with the piece, the frontal hair line is terrific to utilize with the tape. There is also an area on either side of the middle part where the hair line is naturally curved which is commonly referred to as the recession area. Just pull the wig forward slightly and adhere to this area.

Sex, Wigs and Whispers

Before placing the wig directly onto your head make sure you have lined it up correctly. Once you are sure of its positioning, press wig down onto your scalp and hold for 3 seconds. If you have to move it to a different position, do it quickly and immediately press down again.

Aside from regular wig tape, there are several stronger tapes on the market that range from CreatedHair Water Wig™ special tape used for all exercise as well as daily wear, and for those who are looking for added security especially when dealing with perspiration, to those made to adhere longer which are commonly used with bonded pieces.

With the Water Wig™ special tape you should be able to get 2 wears out of the normal wear; one day with 'wet' wear. You can also reactivate the tape by dabbing a small amount of alcohol on it.

When removing all tape, make sure to brush away any hair that may have stuck to tape, then quickly remove tape. If you don't remove the tape, and keep adding more tape on top of it, your own body temperature will cause tape to melt and it will be difficult to remove later on. If this happens, you can go into any beauty supply and ask for wig glue remover.

Dab a little remover onto a Q-tip and rub the remainder of the tape off the wig. Dab with a clean dry cloth towel or paper towel and then reapply tape.

WHAT TO DO WHEN YOU HAVE NO TAPE

There have been times when I have been without my tape and actually used strong scotch tape or packing tape turned inside out and connected to make a circle. Although it didn't hold very long and had to be changed often, it helped until I could get my hands on some wig tape.

Keep in mind that most regular wig tape does not stick well to silicone or certain types of polyurethane material, or the material used in many areas of a wig ranging from the edges of a wig to the temples, sideburns and nape areas.

Red Tape, Ad Mat 3M Tape, Lace Tape or Water Wig™ Tape will work better with these materials. Sewing tape tabs as explained above is recommended if needed.

THE DO'S AND DON'TS FOR WOMEN OF COLOR

And now some advice from Emmy Nominated Celebrity Stylist: Kathleen Leonard. Thanks for the info, Kath!

What are some of the biggest challenges African American women have with their hair?

Hair at the nape can get tangled especially from perspiration. It's also a challenge keeping the hair style, as it reverts back to its original natural texture when the hair is exposed to moisture, salt, or perspiration.

Solution

When that happens it's best to use a relaxer. However, if not done correctly or too often, it will dry the hair and result in hair breakage, so it's important to keep it conditioned.

To make it easier, Kathleen suggests:

- Find a hairstyle that fits your lifestyle.
- Wear a wig so you don't stress your own hair out.

Best Shampoo

"Wen Conditioning Cleanser"

Sulfate-Free moisturizing shampoo; "Shea Moisture Shampoo and Conditioner" works well. You can cleanse just with conditioner and it will work fine.

Tools – What to Use and Not to Use

Best Comb – Wide Tooth Comb

Best Brush – Paddle Brush

Pressing Hair

When pressing hair; always use a white piece of tissue to test the heat level of the comb to avoid burning the hair.

Heated Pressing Comb

Never go higher than 415 degrees to flat iron. Baby Bliss flat iron works well.

Oils to Use

- Moroccan oil
- Argan oil
- Olive oil
- Mineral Oil

5-6 drops for thick hair per section – 1-2 times a week

Intimacy

"Men understand from their Mama – there is No touching the hair without permission."

"If your hair is a reflection of fabulous playin', you can flatten it out afterwards.

"Aside from wrapping or braiding your hair, placing a silk cap over your hair is always a first choice.

"Using a satin pillow case will reduce static from the piece.

"Cotton pillow cases absorb the oils out of the hair leaving it dry where satin pillow cases do not.

Kathleen has been working with me for 8 years. She's talented, patient, inspirational and has been wonderful with my clients that are going through cancer treatment and Alopecia.

Being Caucasian, I was curious as to the differences in hair issues between the two races, so we sat down and she explained a bit to me. I was intrigued...she said,

"It takes so long for the hair to be styled, most African American women don't like to go into the water because it causes the hair to revert back its natural hair style or worse, lose the style they just received. It is for this reason that they'll wait until they see their stylist to get their hair washed and have their braids put in or replaced, which explains why women of color will always shower with a cap.

"Most black men say they don't like women with extensions or weaves, but at the same time are turned on by them, which is one of the reasons why black women love to get them.

"Women of color will always have a cute little satin scarf that they'll tie around their hair to keep it in tact to prevent their hair from getting tangled or destroying the style that's she just sat for

Sex, Wigs and Whispers

hours getting done. It's accepted by black men, as this is what their mothers and grandmothers have always done for centuries.

"In sports, 99% of the time African American women will braid their hair.

"If they've had their hair pressed or had thermal straightening, most black women will avoid rain, aggressive activities and sports – all so they can save their hair.

"The average time for pressing is 1-3 weeks but will largely depend on the location you live in. The least amount of time a black woman will spend in the beauty parlor is 25-45 minutes. However the average time in the beauty parlor is 2-4 hours."

- Weaves: 4-9 hours, every 2-3 months. Avg. cost $125 to as much as $1,000

- Braids: 1- 16 hours depending on the type of braid they desire

- Micro braids can take up to 16 hours and cost between $200-$700 dollars

- Corn Rows take 20 min to 2 hours and will cost $25-$85 dollars

- A touch up or relax and style can take anywhere from 2 1/2 hours to 4 and cost $45-125

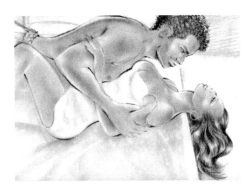

If an African American woman has recently gotten her hair done, it is not uncommon during lovemaking for her to hang her head off the bed to avoid matting and tangling.

THE WORLD OF WIGS

In the world of wigs, it's important to understand what you are wearing and the differences between a human hair and synthetic wigs.

The difference is vast in quality, maintenance and price. Human hair is 100% natural. It is literally hair that has been taken off someone's head. In Europe women stand in line to offer their hair as buyers pay top dollar. Hindu pilgrims have donated their hair at holy temples throughout Southern India for centuries in an attempt to purify themselves and repay debt to their gods.

Synthetic is made of several different fibers including nylon. Both can look fabulous.

Human hair calls for more maintenance when washing where synthetic fibers often hold their shape after drying naturally. Keep in mind, that the better the synthetic fiber the stronger the "memory stay".

You can use heat products on human hair where most synthetic fibers, aside from some heat resistant fibers or CreatedHair.com Active Wigs, will burn from heating instruments. (See *Dealing with Frizz* section on page 274)

I'll let you in on a little secret: no matter what anyone may tell you, the truth is, the cut is what can make or break a good wig. Since wigs do not breathe or have natural oils like human follicles, it takes a very experienced stylist to the cut the piece correctly. It's challenging to find stylists who are comfortable working with wigs and in my experience, even fewer stylists really know how to work with synthetics.

After many years of searching I have found the best and most creative stylists who understand the art of wigs, but believe me it has been a painful process. Plenty of good wigs have been ruined by stylists who thought they knew what they were doing, only to find out how different and very difficult the technique can be.

When looking for a wig stylist, make sure you ask the stylist:

- How long they have been cutting wigs?

- Are they comfortable working on both synthetic and human hair?

- If not both, which do they prefer working on?

- Ask to see before and after photos of their work.

- Make sure you tell them to take their time; you don't want to rush the cut. After all, it won't grow back!

- Don't hesitate to honor yourself here. Stick to your guns.

AFFIRMATION

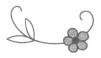

*I make the time to investigate the right stylist for my needs.
I no longer make hasty decisions either out of fear
of not finding any other stylist, or out of the need
to get my wig done at that exact moment.
I made an important investment.
I honor the time it takes to finish it correctly.*

PART

8

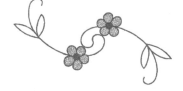

Life's Surprises

Finding Bill

*"Take the first step in faith.
You don't have to see the whole staircase.
Just take the first step."*

Martin Luther King, Jr.

How many of you are looking for Mr. or Ms. Right? How many of you – work all week, too tired to go out, don't go to bars, not comfortable meeting at a gym – not looking our best or having that wonderful fragrance about us? *Am I ringing a bell here? Ahh, another thing we have in common.*

I had decided it was time to find my life mate; I wasn't too sure about marriage after my last engagement ten years ago, but I definitely knew that I was ready to find the man that I was going to live my next fifty years or so with – if I'm lucky. Not knowing where to begin looking, I decided to go on the Internet and try online dating. My sister knew a lot about Internet dating, and immediately discouraged me, claiming it to be mostly shallow, superficial and that I'll never attract someone spiritual like me.

"On these matchmaking sites Amy, guys you like, 45-55 years old, are on there mostly for 'Sport Sex' and will never go for a girl your age, he's searching for a 28-32 year old, not a 48 year old. And these girls make it their career to look good for the man of their dreams. You're too deep; they're all shallow and thin and, well... you know you've got a weight issue. And I'm sorry honey, if you look at their photos – I just don't want to see you hurt – but most have beautiful hair. You'll never have a chance. The men on these sites can be rude and I don't want to see you get hurt."

So I turned to my sister, who I love dearly, but can be a 'know-it-all' and said,

"I appreciate your point of view; however, I believe what Mom always says: 'What you think is what you create.' And, regardless of what you feel about my online hunting, I know that I am 'already' attracting the perfect man who is going to adore my 'Jewish' butt and thighs, love the same songs, speak the same language, connect to my spirit and... he's going to love my bald head. Trust me; by the fall I will be with my perfect soul mate because that's what I will create."

Sex, Wigs and Whispers

Since most of these sites offer over six million members, I figured it was simply a numbers game and sooner or later I would find my life mate; so, I decided to give it a shot and take a chance. We are all evolving, and at different stages in our life we call for different needs, and if there is one thing you can be sure of in life – it's that nothing stays the same; so we have to keep ourselves open to change. However, I was surprised at the amount of opposition I received from those closest to me.

My Public Relations agent had an interesting reaction, "Amy, how could you do this? You can't be serious! You're just going to hang all your dirty laundry for thousands of people to see when I work my butt off creating an air of mystery around you."

After Reviewing several profiles on this matchmaking site, I decided to take a different approach than all the rest of the female profiles that advertised with, *"I want a man who likes to take long romantic sunset walks, loves a girl in jeans by day, but looks great in a gown."* Blah, Blah,Blah; BORING!

Mine was a bit more to the point:

The man I would be drawn to would be conscious, (which meant spiritual – whereas some 'non – contenders' – the operative word here – thought it meant awake and not sleeping!)

He would be aware of his body temple and he would embrace chivalry and not resent it.

At 8 years old my father told me, "you'll never hold onto a man from a can." So he sent me to my Aunt's twice a month to learn how to cook incredible gourmet meals without using a recipe. So, if you're not into entertaining, I suggest you turn the page.

I believe dogs are people with fur. I've learned it's best to date those with the same sensitivities; so, if you're not on the same page then I suggest you move on.

The man I would be drawn to has found his passion in life and is not afraid to live it.

Oh and by the way, I'm looking for a real man, so boys need not apply.

The amazing response: all except a few were looking for a serious relationship. Then one day, I received a note from this man named Bill stating that he had received my information from the site we were both on, whose 'computer system' felt that based on our profiles, we would be compatible. He was really cute. My first reaction was, *"Really? So you had to wait for someone to send you this? You didn't find me yourself?!"* Augh – the 'ego' can be soooo interesting.

My ego and fear had a way of running together creating doubts in me – causing me to misinterpret him. After a bit of email correspondence we decided to speak on the phone. Everything was going great until *finally* he says, (and I say 'finally,' because I knew this moment would come),

"What's your full name; your last name Amy?"

Oh, No! Now, he's going to Google me and he'll know! At least, I wanted him to get to know me first before having him find out about my secret. I needed him to feel who I was first; instead of him possibly running away. I was too unfamiliar with him and didn't know how he'd react.

I responded,

"Amy G_{innum}" ***(making sure to swallow the last part)***

He said, "What was that? Sorry, I didn't get it."

Sex, Wigs and Whispers

"Amy G<small>innum</small>" *I repeated.*

He said, "Oh, it must be this phone; I'm sorry, I still didn't get that."

I finally blurted out, "GIBSON, AMY GIBSON!"

To which he said "Oh wait a minute; there's someone at my door. I'll call you back."

So I waited a few minutes and my heart started to beat rapidly. I was starting to feel the anxiety, so I called my Mom.

"Ma! I don't think this one is going to work. He's Googling me right now, I know it! It's over!"

My heart was now racing and I began to cry; *I'm sure he found out who I am and everything about my hair loss, and he's not going to want me. I'm going to end up alone, Mom! I like this guy.* I was hysterical now; the more I thought about it, the harder my tears flowed. Then suddenly... the phone rang. I quickly cleared my throat and like the chameleon I had become during my acting years, snapped back to reality, took a breath, picked up that phone, and said with the sexiest voice,

"Hellloo."

"SO! I'm on your site and these wigs are fabulous! You look great. Which one of these pictures are really you?"

Without missing a beat through all my nerves I said,

"All of them."

He said, "That is soo cool."

"YES! Whew! Thank God this guy has substance. Loove it!"

So we set a time to meet.

We both arrived for tea and the chemistry was awesome.

He was even more handsome in person. His cool Prada pewter colored sunglasses blended in with his salt and pepper hair that glistened in the sun (which I love, especially with green eyes and his were gorgeous).

After a moment, I took a breath and looked at him and said, "So I have to tell you something right now."

His eyes said "Uh, Oh."

And without thinking, the blunt Sagittarius in me blurted out,

"I lied about my age." To which he quickly responded,

"So did I."

We cracked up laughing. I thought, 'Hmmmm, this could be a definite contender.' I was right; he was deep and didn't care about my baldness. To him, I was and still am truly beautiful – with or without hair, regardless of my weight fluctuations. Hair has nothing to do with my essence, which is what he was and still is, most drawn to.

Little did I know a matchmaking computer would get it right! We were like two peas in a pod! We both practice the same Spiritual beliefs and even belong to the same Spiritual center! We're both in health care, both helping cancer patients worldwide and with a symbiotic mission in life. *What are the chances of that...* Thank you Spirit! What a great man you helped me manifest.

1½ years later we moved in together. The proposal was a complete surprise, with all the romance you could dream of... Yes, we got married and it is wonderful. And he was worth the wait.

To this day he kisses my scalp each night before I go to bed.

Sex, Wigs and Whispers

So just remember – the next time someone says you can't do something; that you're too old, too fat, too thin, not enough hair, not smart enough, wrong ethnicity or why Mr. or Ms. Right isn't out there – you just tell them, "Thank you for your concern – but, "What I believe – I create!"

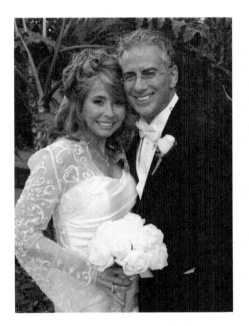

AFFIRMATION

I am fully supported everywhere I stand. I no longer need anyone's approval to move forward with things in life that I believe are correct. I no longer need to question myself, as I have the inner guidance to know what is right for me, for my heart and for my needs and follow that with the utmost faith. I draw the perfect people into my life who are accepting, truthful, unconditional, loving, generous, supportive, funny, non-judgmental, and totally supportive of my passions in life.

Sex, Wigs and Whispers

Bye Bye Brows

"Always be a first rate version of yourself and not a second rate version of someone else."

Judy Garland

This is such an interesting time for me right in the midst of the home stretch of my book, heading towards the finish line. Out of nowhere, I have all of a sudden started going into Alopecia Universalis[1]. **I'm beginning to lose all my body hair!** Never – ever did I expect this. I just always thought my totalis[1] that I had lived with for over 25 years was where it would end. *I guess I was wrong – another one of life's curves to deal with...*

A more intensely stressful time in recent months may have triggered it; although I'm always stressed.

I work often seven days a week; regularly go to sleep late (sometimes 2 am and I wake up at 7 am to get to work). I love what I do, but it is stressful helping my beautiful clients walk through this process with confidence and grace, helping them find peace of mind at his time, especially those who are fighting cancer. In addition to writing, I've been getting The ResQ Bag™ (the first in a line of wig accessories to come) to market in the midst of production dealing with factories on the other side of the globe, while still producing, writing and hosting a web-based television show: "Don't Wig Out!" On top of that, my little dachshund is going into heat for the first time! It's a lot for one person, along with trying to be a good a stepmom and new wife, while constantly reminding myself to stay grateful for it all...

What's been so fascinating for me is that this is the first time in a long time that I've had to actually deal with my hair loss situation. What I mean is, I had developed a rhythm, I finally had gotten a handle on this ride and have been able to steer pretty steadily, avoiding the deadly curves but taking the bumps pretty well, while continuing to move at a consistent speed – safely. I think it's called unconscious competence.

. . . .

1   total scalp hair loss

Sex, Wigs and Whispers

However I feel like now, I've hit a sudden break in the road and I'm unsure where to go or how I'll get to wherever this journey is taking me safely.

It's bringing back a lot of painful memories from when I first started losing my hair and all the fears and insecurities about my looks that would live in me before I found some relief from the cortisone shots I took which, for almost 17 years allowed me to keep my hair loss in check. Until the last big crash of course – when after having a reaction to the steroids, I stopped treatment and lost all my hair in just three weeks.

I'm flashing on my entree into the journey of hair loss and wigs and what I went through in learning how to live with them, which was a constant maze of fear and confusion. The more confused I got, the angrier and more freaked out I became over my hair loss. Then, of course, are all the crazy experiences that followed which forced me to learn how to lie really well to keep my secret. It's amazing how our survival instincts will take over when called upon. All of this has led to my developing the tips I'm sharing with you.

And now, after I have it all organized – no eyebrows or lashes? The two things that frame my face most? *Really! What the hell am I supposed to do with that! How does a woman live with that? How do I keep from feeling 'less than'?*

I still want to look beautiful. I want to look beautiful for me, for my husband, for my clients, for my business and to help me propel forward in my life with my mission. I need my brows to make me feel complete and to fulfill my dreams for what I want to do in this life and for so many others who are also living with this crazy condition. But how can I do this authentically for others if I can't get a handle on this myself first?

For the first time – in a long time, I'm really feeling like a deep layer of my sensuality and my sexuality has suddenly been stripped from me and from my soul. I am vividly feeling like I first did and the fears I had of nobody liking me anymore, friends turning away from me because they had no idea how to deal with me, or my tears. It's bringing back painful memories of when I was so scared from being ousted from the entertainment industry and feeling so very alone on this wild journey.

I feel I'll look like an alien without eyebrows. I'll look really weird. I won't be pretty. I have so many fears around what's going to happen. I've stayed up all last week, barely being able to get to sleep for even a 3 hours a night. I've been crying, grieving, staring at myself a lot in the mirror, comparing photos of myself and judging my butt, my thighs, my face, everything. I just haven't been able to stop dissecting myself. I feel overwhelmed – again.

My husband must be so sick of it, although he is so sweet and giving, he would never say a word. He'll listen to the same rhetoric over and over again and say, "Honey it's not that bad, you're beautiful! I really feel your lashes and brows will grow back." Maybe they will… But even though I know he means it – I also imagine he's saying that so I don't lose it!

Now all I can do is my best to stay positive – and calm – because I live in a proactive world and refuse to feel like a victim in this life or to this condition! I'm just going to have to keep from dwelling too long in this fear. I'm going to have push myself to move through this; but, there are days when it just can be so hard.

One part of me knows I'm living through it, regardless of how depressed I feel and that it will all be fine, while the other part feels completely out of control and can't stop crying. It feels like it's there still bubbling right below my feet just waiting to rise up.

Sex, Wigs and Whispers

Now, I feel like I'm accepting what is. If the rest of my eyebrow leaves me, so be it, at least there's brow tattooing and I've been trying out and learning about all the great brow pencils there are on the market. Some are really fabulous. It's a bit of a learning curve, but I'm getting the hang of it. And to my surprise, I'm actually having fun experimenting. Of course, I have become obsessed. *I must have purchased every pencil from every maker in every store! From drug stores to the mall, I've learned to use them all.*

I decided to go into Nordstoms and get a lesson from one of their trained makeup artists. But there were so many; how was I going to find the right one to show me how to deal with this and help me create my new look? So I parked and did the only thing I knew to do in times like this; I closed my eyes and went into prayer; *"Ok Mom, lead me to the right person, and quickly please. I don't have a lot of time between clients and I need to get a handle on this, the clock's ticking – please Mom help me so I can feel myself again."*

As I walked in, Nordstroms was packed. After all, it was 3PM on a Saturday! I thought, *"am I crazy to do this right now! There are at least four makeup artists rushing around helping customers with purchases, a couple more who are in the middle of doing a customers' personal makeup. How the hell am I going to find one who really knows about brows?"* From my days on set, I knew it was a specialty. Just at that moment, a beautiful woman walked up to me and asked if she could help me. I told her,

Oh Thank you, I am trying to find a makeup artist who really knows about eyebrows. At which point she hands me her card – which says "Brow Specialist"! Go Mom!

Kristi generously spent two hours teaching me about shape and technique and helped me so much, that upon leaving I felt like a piece of me had returned. Even if it were only until I washed my face.

I have found that DEFINE-A-BROW® by Maybelline with a flat end and small comb at the tip is best. The flat end makes it look more like a smudge than a deep line that comes from using a pointed pencil. Yet it still allows you to achieve a more pointed direct line if needed. And the comb adds to a more natural look. Just 'lightly' run the comb over your brows after you've finished your drawing. Using a slightly darker shade in a pointed pencil can work if you lightly place a stroke of a hair here and there to give a bit of definition and realistic look. The key here is keeping a light hand when drawing all brows. If you feel it's too challenging to get the shape correct, there are wonderful eyebrow stencils to help guide your hands that are available at most beauty supplies and on line. I suggest that in the beginning you get the ones that come closest to the brows you used to have. You can get creative later. Luckily after Kristi's lessons, and years of helping my clients draw on their brows using stencils and brows free-hand, it's seems to be easier for me to draw my own without the use of stencils.

If you're comfortable, keep in mind that this is the time you can change your look as well, so get a few and play with it.

Alright, so if I have no more arm hair, underarm hair, leg hair, very little eyebrows and no eyelashes or pubic hair. So be it. The hell with it all! At least I can wear lashes and I can learn how to do my brows so well they will become a fun hobby instead of a hardship. I've got to stay grateful for everything. It's the only way to find peace.

Sex, Wigs and Whispers

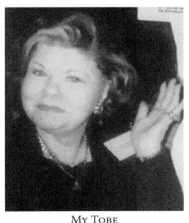

My Tobe

I can hear my Mom's words from years ago bellowing in my head,

"Amy – you're so lucky, God gave you a beautiful face, a sharp mind and most of all a beautiful deep soul. You're so lucky you can see – you can hear, you can walk – you have two breasts – cherish those things. Be thankful. Hair – ahh, you can replace it with a thousand gorgeous wigs, but you can't replace your soul. Remember, women are amazing beings. We can move mountains with our minds. If you're going to hold on to anything, hold on to that."

And so this is where I am today. However I told my husband he needs to shoot the cover of the book while I still have some brows... who knows, we'll see if I still have them by the time we get there.

AFFIRMATION

My Condition has no control of my soul.
My 'condition' is just that – nothing more.
It does not dictate my humor, my wit,
my ability to love myself or others.
It has no effect on my level of depth
or my ability to be normal like other women.

Today – I make the choice to move beyond appearances
and know the truth of my true being
and live only in that reality.

Eyebrows

Forgiveness

*"Forgiveness is unlocking the door
to set someone free and realizing
you were the prisoner."*

Max Lucado

This is a chapter I never would've imagined writing while doing this book. But as with everything in life, the one thing you can depend on – is change.

I hadn't spoken to my father for the two years since my wedding; when he chose to create another emotionally abusive episode. I had finally decided after making excuses for him my entire life, that to write him a letter was what I should do and ended our relationship. Until recently, when my sister called me with news of his possible passing, and suggested I meet with him one last time to say whatever it was that was lingering or required closure for both of us. The truth is, he has always been terribly frightened of death. Something I have never had a fear of; instead, I've harbored an 'intuitive knowing' since a young child of what is waiting for all of us on the other side, a large part of that being love.

However, I have always considered his fear to be the result of the guilt he has deep in his heart for how he abused me, and who knows how many others; and thus, is scared to death he's going to Hell, fearing all that awaits such a guest.

When my sister broached the subject of his molestation on my behalf, I was told he fluffed it off as, "Ah, that was nothing." Needless to say, I was infuriated, only adding more difficulty to this last meeting.

I found myself at an emotional crossroads; part of me could have cared less about his well-being or fears, for I had shed many tears in therapy working through all that and uncovering what I learned was necessary for me to love myself again. I went through hell to progress in my life to a more positive place and have healthy relationships. In my mind and heart, on the deepest level I had moved on, period.

Sex, Wigs and Whispers

I had vowed NO more Abuse, No more Sickness. No more Tears! Yet, the other part of me knew that once he was gone, there would be no way for me to say the things I felt I needed to say, thereby achieving real and total closure. I knew I was not doing this for him. I was doing it for me. No hanging threads left behind. I needed to let him know it was okay to go now and that I forgave him so he could go in peace. And I could truly put my feelings to rest.

Much easier said than done as that meant I truly had to do just that; forgive him on the deepest level. I wondered if I was capable. *Could I really let go of all the pain, hurt, judgment and intense anger? Not in 2 hours, no way; 2 years... maybe.* I had no idea what I was in for with this forthcoming experience, but the one thing I was sure of was that I had to move through this intense episode – regardless of the attachment to those old emotions that I held on to for so long – again, for my own well-being.

On the 2½ hour drive down to his home, many things ran through my mind; from anger and resentment, to disturbing flashbacks. It brought me back to the time I was in development on a television series I had created for TriStar. My Father had invited me to lunch at his home in San Diego. It was one of the best times we had shared in a couple of years. We talked a lot about business, for which he had always offered great guidance and laughed a lot. But then, suddenly in the midst of this wonderful energy, he excused himself from the table for which I thought was to use the bathroom; but instead, was faced with something bizarre: he returned to the table with a shoe box filled with papers and proceeded to tell me,

"You know, Ame, over the years you certainly have been given a lot. Yup – I certainly have spent a lot of money since you were a child. Now I know with your new contact you'll be getting $20,000 – $30,000 a month, and I was wondering if you could reimburse me for a few things."

My first thought was confusion. He proceeded to mention bills as far back as my braces at age eight and all the dental work he had to pay for, to insignificant bills that are the norm for any parent to cover. I was appalled, starkly clear of his intention for this lunch.

"First of all," I shot back, "I haven't made a cent yet as this contract is based on only 'if and when' the show sells. Aside from that, I've been working for free at the studio for eight months, getting it ready to present to the networks. That's how it works as an independent producer. However with that said, I can't believe you would bring up some of these costs which are simple things that any parent covers when bringing up a child."

Now, I was furious as his self-absorbed and skewed thinking was sinking in even more. I continued, "You know, I have always been incredibly generous with this entire family. Whenever anyone has ever needed anything I have been there and never hesitated in sending money: for the house taxes, the private schools, cars, even your three hair transplants. Thousands and thousands of dollars:, and I've never asked for it to be returned. I have just given from my heart. It's who I am. I understand if you need the money, but the way you have gone about this today is disgusting, dysfunctional and dishonest!" I took a breath – looked him straight in the eye, and said, "So, let me ask you something – when you knocked my Mother up, was there any responsibility you took on after that?"

Sex, Wigs and Whispers

I got up abruptly, left and proceeded to drive home for two and a half hours in tears. It would be two years before we would speak again. And of course when we did, nothing was ever discussed, nor did he apologize.

As I continued my drive to his home, other flashbacks would come to mind from his supportive moments, to the beautiful times we did share, through the years of emotional outbursts, countless lies and sick behavior. I felt waves of nausea, the type that would strike me years prior that would repeatedly get stuck in my throat; I had to breathe through it until it passed. I'd put on an upbeat Pharell song to break the moment and get me in a better mood, but after the song finished, feelings of great sadness would return. Some were conscious, some unconscious. I had a short discussion with my therapist on the phone, who was kind enough to talk me through this anxiety, in between handling all her clients, which seemed to help for a short time.

I practiced aloud what I was going to say when we would meet. *Do I hug him or keep my distance?* I knew that regardless of any rehearsed monologue, what was most important for me was to stay present and deal with the Devil that I was about to meet... for the last time, in this life.

She told me he was ill and could barely speak or stand. However, in the last 25 years it had become clear what a hypochondriac he was; lying about so many things that I never knew how to assess what was real with him.

I arrived on his street and pulled over. I found myself rushing to put my lashes on perfectly, fixing my makeup to carve whatever fat I was trying to hide in my cheeks and color them to create the jawline he always loved and approved of.

Forgiveness

I knew what I was doing consciously and at the same time felt like I was watching myself from above on automatic.

I met my sister and we drove 1 block to his home. She told me that he had prepared being "up" for me the entire day! I thought, *'Oh God what's that gonna' look like?'*

As I walked in, I saw a frail thin man sitting up in bed with missing teeth; something he would never allow to happen in his recent years. He said, "Amm – my Amy; Let me look at you – you look so young."

I walked over and gave him a kiss on the cheek and a light hug and thought, *'Well, I had gotten my first star of the evening.'*

He asked how I was and I kept it light and safe at first by talking about business. I brought him up to date about my new ResQ Bag™ which was entering the market in 2 weeks on the #1 wig retailer website in the world and all the other wonderful business I had at the moment. Then he asked about Bill and the kids. "You got married – how was it?"

I thought, *'Oh oh, he's getting personal – here we go...'*

I wasn't surprised that he swept such a life changing event under the carpet. After all, I disowned him prior to my wedding and had my favorite cousin Jerry give me away instead; a decision I struggled with, but felt I had to do for my own well-being. I was sure he felt something, but he was keeping it safe. I had learned when in doubt, mirror the person you're with. I did just that and replied,

"It was beautiful Dad – would you like to see?"

After showing him lots of photos, I found it par for the course he never asked why he wasn't invited, why I disappeared, or who walked me down the aisle in his place; and wasn't willing to take any responsibility for his ugly disgusting behavior prior to my wedding. Of course, being in Ladies Retail for so many years, he jumped at the chance to really review the design lines of my dress and what he seemed to be most interested in.

But then again, I have to remember; he does have a bit of Dementia, or is it likely straight up denial? Perhaps an unanswerable question since he always acted out of control, with incredible bouts of anger and bursts of defiance. Including betraying anyone that befriended him. At the same time, the paradox is that he was also very generous, and at times a very supportive father; especially when it came to my acting career and personal aspirations, which made it all the more confusing for me.

So in the end, maybe it's simply dysfunction.

He loved my ring and immediately reached for his jewelry loop that he purchased while taking his Gemology course, to check the facets of the diamond and then gave me his approval. He loved the bridesmaid's dresses, the material, colors, the event's decor etc. and of course, thought Bill looked smashing. We discussed my new dog, my kids and a bit more business, and then it was time; I looked at him, took a long beat and said...

"Dad, I came here to let you know I forgive you, and its okay to go now. You can go in peace"

No reply.

I felt my heart start to beat in that same way it would when I heard his footsteps before coming into my room.

Forgiveness

Still no reply. Silence.

I was determined to wait it out.

Finally, he responded,

"WELL YOU KNOW AMY, THERE'S THAT ISSUE ABOUT THE $10,000 I LOANED YOU IN '98 ON THAT REAL ESTATE DEAL THAT YOU HAVE NEVER RETURNED."

I was taken aback. *Was it his dementia talking? Nah, he's pretty lucid.* It took me moment to catch my breath.

"I had forgotten all about that," I said, with no small amount of sadness for an entirely missed life-moment. "You're right, I guess I got so caught up with dealing with life and survival while building a business from the trunk of my car, focusing on my client's needs, making a name for myself with my new designs, and dealing with health issues", (some as a result from his abuse) I literally forgot. I am so sorry."

I could have reminded him of all the finances I generously covered when they were strapped, which was their responsibility, but it never came to my mind. Not until I was driving back the next day. All I could say was that I was sorry. It was most unfortunate that I never got that in return.

"I will pay you back I promise."

I said I had to go, gave him a kiss, told him I loved him and left.

It was a long, very sad drive home.

At least I am clear in my heart now. I am able now to wish him well. I've become wise about my own wholeness.

I am at peace, for I know three things: 1) Desperate people do desperate things; it doesn't mean that they're conscious of what they're doing during the act– which is also what makes this type of person so dangerous to be around. 2) People do the best they can with the tools given them. 3) For me to move on and to truly find peace within myself with this process, I must learn to forgive the *doer*, which doesn't mean I have to forgive the *deed*.

I don't expect this process to be completed overnight as I'm still processing this, especially through the writing of this book. I know there are more positive qualities about him that I will genuinely miss. I'm glad I went, glad I saw him and glad I was able to kiss him goodbye.

As of this writing he is still alive. As I said, he is having a hard time letting himself go. I pray he finds peace within his heart, so when it is his time to cross the veil he can go without so much fear.

AFFIRMATION

I always know when I have had enough;
when my heart, mind and soul can bear no more.
I listen, follow and most of all, honor myself in my process.

Epilogue

Dear Reader,

My intention with this book was to first give some helpful and useful tips that I've used myself and felt would benefit others. However, while working on it, other issues kept coming up that I felt were important to share, so I put them in.

I hope through this book you've gotten some solutions and insight for whatever you wished to learn or overcome. I hope you laughed, and I hope it helped you remember who you are, which is magnificent – hair or no hair. Finally, I hope it will help you reconnect with your light, if you've lost it.

We all have a story, make yours one you can dance to.

Thank you for allowing me to share mine with you.

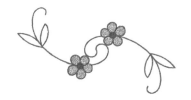

Appendices

Appendix A

Your physician will provide you with a prescription for your wig known in medical terms as a, "Full Cranial Hair Prosthesis." Be sure to call your insurance provider and find out if your policy includes this coverage (including the specific reimbursement amount and number of wigs).

There should be a section under "covered expenses" relating to prostheses, prosthetic devices or medical durable equipment. Most insurance companies don't spell out exclusions so pay attention to the actual coverage.

Be sure to write down the date, first name, last name and phone number/extension of the customer service representative who provides you with the information, along with the detailed coverage information.

Save this information should you need it for future reference.

It is very important to provide your insurance provider with the "procedure code" for a full cranial hair prosthesis which looks similar to this: A9282. However there are different codes for each condition and they sometimes change per year, so be sure to ask your doctor's office for your specific procedure code.

After you have purchased your wig, the salon will provide you with a purchase receipt that you will need to submit to your insurance provider for possible direct reimbursement back to you.

Be sure you make a photocopy of the cranial prosthesis prescription for your files and submit the original along with the purchase receipt for your wig and any necessary insurance form they require.

Be sure to mail the necessary paperwork described above directly to your insurance provider via U.S. Post Office Certified Mail – Return Receipt. Keep the green postcard return receipt you will receive by U.S. mail once the paperwork has been delivered to your insurance company.

Remember to keep the photocopy of your purchase receipt, the prescription and any reimbursement form you submit to your insurance provider.

Be sure when completing the insurance company's reimbursement form that you indicate reimbursement should be sent to you directly.

Always call 3-4 days after sending to confirm they have received it and keep the name of the person who signed for it.

If you have any questions, I will do my best to help in any way I can. So send me your questions to:

Book@Createdhair.com

Appendix B

GLOSSARY FOR INTELLIGENT DECISIONS

Wig: A general term used to describe different types of products to replace hair.

Ventilation: The art of sewing strands of either human hair or synthetic hair into the base of the wig cap.

Machine-Made Wigs: Wigs that are made from wefts of hair that are sewn on by machine.

Hairpiece: Hairpieces are worn in place of growing hair. They are partial pieces or add-ons used to create additional volume or length to existing hair.

Custom Wig: A custom wig that is made to your particular specifications; the manufacturer will use any combination of hair fiber, cap, styles, color to get you exactly what you want in a wig that looks and feels like you.

Custom Quality Specialty Wig: A high quality wig or cranial prosthesis that is designed with base materials so that the cap may be altered to achieve an excellent fit. It is very comparable to some special order custom hair pieces.

Daily Wear Cranial Prosthesis: This is a type of cranial prosthesis that can be removed each day. It can be secured with a special tape that can be removed at the end of the day. These prostheses will not require any type of bonding material.

Cap: The base material that gives the wig its shape and a base to attach hair to.

C3 Construction: Construction utilizing the 3 C's: **Cool**: lets your scalp breathe; **Comfortable**: constructed with new, softer and lighter materials; **Capless**: so lightweight you won't even know it's there.

Sex, Wigs and Whispers

STANDARD CAP: A standard cap is the most common and most affordable cap design. The layers of hair are open-wefted in the back and sides to allow for ventilation and have a closed lace layer at the crown.

The hair at the crown is often lightly teased or crimped so you can not see down through the cap. This type of cap often gives the hair a natural lift at the crown for volume. However this cap can be a bit heavier and get warmer to wear this being less comfortable than a cap with a monofilament top.

CAPLESS WIG: Very similar to the standard cap design; however, it does not have the closed lace layer at the crown. It is open-wefted in the back, sides and crown. This allows for maximum ventilation and for the ability to pull your own hair through. It is also the lightest weight cap you can purchase.

ADJUSTABLE CAP: A wig cap construction with adjustable tabs that extend from the crown to the nape of the wig cap. Average wig cap can either be adjusted to a smaller or larger cap size.

MEMORY CAP: A wig cap that replaces the wide stretch lace used in most of today's wigs with a thinner, more resilient stretch material that actually molds to the shape of the head for a lighter, more secure fit.

MONOFILAMENT/MONO-TOP WIG: A Monofilament/Mono-Top Wig refers to fine, breathable nylon or silk mesh with hairs individually hand-knotted into the mesh. It disappears against the scalp allowing natural skin tone and appears as a natural looking part giving it more versatility in styling. It is recommended for hair loss patients and allows comfort and excellent ventilation.

LACE FRONT: A wig made with a mesh insert in the front into which individual hairs are hand-tied.It creates a realistic looking hairline. When properly worn with a special adhesive, it is almost undetectable that it is not the wearer's own growing hair. They are more expensive and difficult to manage and do not last as long as other wigs.

VELVET FRONT: A small piece of soft, velvety material inserted into the front of a wig to create a more comfortable fit at the hairline.

OPEN WEFTED CAPS: Open wefted caps have a natural skin top that resembles a scalp. From the crown to the nape, there are many wefts (rows of hair) sewn horizontally across from ear to ear.

The area between each weft is open so the cap does not feel as tight on the head. When pinning a wig up, the open wefts allow the pins to go through the cap and be fastened to the hair growing from the head, which assures a firmed hold. The open wefts also allow more ventilation to the scalp.

CLOSE WEFTED CAPS: Closed wefted caps have a natural skin top that resembles a scalp. From the crown to the nape, there is a single piece of stretch material with wefts sewn horizontally across from ear to ear. This cap has a snugger fit and because the single piece of material is completely closed to the head, it prevents hair from the head from coming through. Due to the snug fit, many women wearing wigs for Alopecia or wigs for cancer prefer the closed wefted cap.

VACUUM BASE WIG: A wig designed to stay on by means of suction due to the customized fit.

Sex, Wigs and Whispers

Silicone Lining: Silicone Lining is a comfortable added element of small strips of silicone in key areas in and around the cap to prevent the wig or hair piece from slipping.

Silicone Closed Wefted Cap: Wefted caps with added pieces or lining of silicone that offers the wig wearer the ultimate comfort and security without the use of clips, combs, glues and tapes. This cap is ideal for women suffering from any type of full hair loss.

Skin Top: Gives the illusion of hair growing out of the scalp. This look can be achieved through French-part ventilation or polyurethane material.

Lace: A base material.

Lace Lip: Narrow bang section of lace material that rests on the forehead, creating a natural hairline.

Ribbon Edge: Material usually doubled over and placed along the outer edge of a lace base.

CREATEDHAIR.COM

Date Needed_____

MEASUREMENTS FOR SPECIAL WIGS

Salon

Client

	Inches
1. Around the head	_____
2. Forehead to nape of neck	_____
3. Ear to ear across forehead	_____
4. Ear to ear over the top	_____
5. Temple to temple around back	_____
6. To nape	_____
7. Behind ear under occipital bone	_____

BEGIN HERE

FOLLOW EVENLY ALL AROUND THE BACK TO THE PLACE YOU BEGAN

DENSITY	High Lights - Low Lights
Light	
Med Light	1/8 1/4 1/2 3/4
Medium	
Heavy	
Very Heavy	

Style	Ventilator:_____
	Total Hours Estimate:
	Total Hours Actual:

348

FITTING SHEET: A process by which to log your measurements: (see opposite page)

CAP SIZES:

PETITE CAP SIZE
The petite cap size is generally the following measurements:

Circumference: Around the Head: 20"

Front to Back: 12 1/8

Ear to Ear: 10 ½

PETITE/AVERAGE CAP SIZE
The petite/average cap size is generally the following measurements:

Circumference: Around the Head: 21¼"

Front to Back: 13 ¾

Ear to Ear: 13 ¼ "

AVERAGE CAP SIZE
The average cap size is generally the following measurements:

Around the Head: 21 ½: 22

Front to Back: 14 ¼: 14 ½

Ear to Ear: 13 ½

AVERAGE/LARGE CAP SIZE
The average/large cap size is generally the following measurements:

Around the Head: 22 ½ ": 23"

Front to Back: 14 ¾: 15

Ear to Ear: 13 ¾: 14

LARGE CAP SIZE

The large cap size is generally the following measurements:

Around the Head: 23 ¼" : 24"

Front to Back: 15 ¼ : 15 ½

Ear to Ear: 14

HUMAN HAIR WIGS: Wigs made of human hair primarily cut in India, China, and parts of Europe which are obtained and contracted through a factory for the specific purpose of making wigs/hairpieces. These wigs can be dyed, permed, and can be carefully used with heating tools.

Wigs made with human hair are very durable; however they require more upkeep than synthetic wigs and must be styled on a regular basis. Generally speaking, although human hair wigs are much heavier than their synthetic counterparts and more expensive, they can actually look and feel more authentic and are worth the money.

UNPROCESSED HAIR: Human hair that has not been chemically treated.

100% EUROPEAN HUMAN HAIR: Is differentiated by genetics rather than geography. It actually refers to Caucasian hair. This is human hair that has retained the cuticle and has undergone a special process to prevent tangling and retain the quality of this extremely fine Caucasian hair. The structure of European hair is a bit finer, flatter and smoother and more desirable. It has a silky texture and comes in all colors from a very pale blonde to jet-black. Because it is less plentiful it is more expensive.

VIRGIN RUSSIAN HAIR: Its fine hair strands, easy movement and amazing durability make this hair the most expensive and sought after in the world. This hair can cost up to $10,000 for a wig 24 inches or longer. It has finer strands. This is an excellent choice for those with thin hair.

VIRGIN HUMAN HAIR WIGS: This is a good but expensive choice if you want the very finest human hair wig. Virgin European hair wigs are high in demand and will range in price from $3000: 8,000 depending on length. They come in short, medium and long styles and are also used in hairpieces and Extensions.

ITALIAN HAIR: Also an expensive choice; on the average Italian hair has a medium texture with a lot of body with the end of the hair being full and blunt. It varies from a slight body wave to a wavy texture. It comes in all colors from a very light almost white to jet-black and will range in price from $2500 to $6,000 depending on length.

CYBERHAIR®: A revolutionary high spun nylon made to look, feel, wash, move and reflect light just like human hair. One cannot tell the difference as the fiber is so real looking. I used this fiber in my international wig line, Amy's Presence®, for my design of the First Women's Swim Wig and The First Women's Intimacy System. This hair does not drag in the water like human hair. It has style memory, so when it dries it reverts back to its original style.

Cyberhair® is a much more sophisticated synthetic which needs moisture and is suggested to be sprayed daily with a Cyberhair® formula called Protection Plus, which will help keep the hair from drying out and getting frizzy like most synthetic fibers. Cyberhair® will range in price from $1450 for stock styles to $4,000 for fully custom made wigs.

HUMAN HAIR BLEND: A combination of human hair and synthetic fiber. The synthetic fiber tends to hold its shape after washing and the human hair looks natural and is more durable. The combination gives the wig more versatility and flexibility in styling. It is usually used in 25%, 35% and 50% ratios to synthetic fibers. However, be careful when using heating tools. I suggest to prevent burning the synthetic hair existing in the blend, you use a temperature of 250 degrees and blow dry on low heat or cool.

REMI/REMY HUMAN HAIR: Refers to human hair (usually Indian in origin) Remy which is less expensive than European, Italian or Russian hair. The hair has been harvested from root to end with the cuticle all going in the same direction that prevents the hair from tangling and is very easy to care for. It may be colored or permed. It is soft and silky and is used for making higher quality wigs, extensions and hairpieces. This quality of hair is often used in cranial prosthesis (wig). It looks very real, however, sometimes can frizz from its texture. Using an ionic straightening iron on the piece will smooth out the frizz.

BABY HAIR: Is the small strands of hair, often curly at the base of the frontal hair line. This hair is often cut from the existing hair in the wig or sewn in to add to a realistic look. Also baby hair can often camouflage the edge of the wig. Occasionally, angora and/or baby Yak hair is used to replicate baby hair. (Refer to Styling section; Shredding)

TEXTURED RELAXED HUMAN HAIR: This is hair that is specially processed and is used in wigs and cranial prosthesis especially designed for most ethnicities including Latina, Persian, and African American Women.

Kanekalon Synthetic Hair Fiber: Kanekalon Fiber is a modacrylic fiber that closely resembles human hair allowing the look, feel and performance characteristics of the real thing.

Synthetic Fiber: There are three types of synthetic fiber used to manufacture wigs, which are polyester, acrylic, and polyvinyl chloride (PVC). They are available in many different lengths and styles.

Synthetic Wigs: Wigs made primarily of modacrylic fibers that have the look and feel of real hair. The fibers have style memory which allows the original styling to be restored in most cases by simply spraying with a water bottle and drying from underneath. They don't fade in color like human hair does.

Part: This is a break where the hair is parted and is usually located at the center or side of the base cap usually 1"- 2" from center. A part can also be referred to as: Left or right just off center, which usually means its 1/4" to 1/2" from center on either side.

Skin Part: Refers to a strip of fabric, usually silk, along the part where the hair is threaded. It gives the appearance of the hair growing directly from the scalp. The part cannot be changed. Wigs with a skin part give you a very natural look.

Simulated Part: A part that is not clearly defined and usually at the center or side of the cap.

Multidirectional/ Multidirectional Part: Higher quality skin top wigs which can be combed or parted in any direction, much like your own hair. It allows you to change the part to right, left or center as desired by wearer.

French Part: French Top Style of ventilation that creates a natural looking skin top for a more natural look. This labor intensive, double ventilation process creates a product that has no returns. Due to the intricate nature of the construction, this style can require more upkeep and maintenance.

Hand-Tied: A term for individual hair fiber that is tied by hand onto the wig cap/base using a single or double knot. Offers styling flexibility and resembles the movement of natural hair.

Honeycomb Wefting: Can be found in either a full or partial hairpiece. Often referred to as an "Integration" piece, it is made with large open holes designed to pull your own hair through.

Add-Ons: Is a partial hair piece: not a full wig; a hairpiece that temporarily attaches either by interlocking combs or butterfly clip to your own hair to add instant length, volume and texture.

Wiglet: A spot enhancer that is designed to work with your own hair to add volume or length in a specific area.

Top of the Head: 'Toppers' as they are often referred to, is a partial piece that fits on the crown to be used to add volume for a fuller look. They come in many length and base sizes.

Fall: Is a partial wig most often used to add length to a style and almost full coverage of the head, while allowing plenty of ventilation and the guarantee of a secure fit. There are three basic types: Full Falls, Headband Falls, Hat Falls:

Full falls allow the wearer's own hair to show at the front and be blended into the hairpiece.

Headband falls or 3/4 wigs are positioned 1" to 1 ½" just behind the front and side hairlines allowing the blending of the front and sides of your hair in with the Fall to create a more voluminous natural looking head of hair. Usually connects easily to your own hair with a series of flex wig combs. It gives a realistic appearance of hair growing directly from the wearer's scalp.

Hat falls are often referred to as "Chemo Cap", have a bare cap on top held together by pieces of elastic in a crisscross design that fit securely on the head where the hair or wefts are attached from the temple down giving the "perfect elusion". This is suggested specifically worn by those with sensitive scalps or seek a lighter feel while wearing a cap or scarf.

INTEGRATION SYSTEM: An integration hair system refers to the type of base material used and is ideal for women (or men) with thinning hair or diffused hair loss like that in Female Pattern Hair Loss. An Integration System allows you to pull your existing, growing hair directly through the unit. This allows you to wear a custom hair replacement system without shaving your head. Your own natural, growing hair is combined with the hair in the system to create a more voluminous and complete head of hair.

WEFTED: A long string of hair fiber attached to a piece of material that is doubled over and sewn closely together.

THIN WEFTING: A weft is a piece of material that has a single of layer of hair fiber sewn into it which is then attached to several other wefts. Many times a wefted cap can result in a lighter, cooler wig. However for those with no hair, especially the challenge in wearing any type of wefted piece, be it extension or wig, is that when the wind blows or you move in a certain direction the wefts will many times show in the back thus exposing your scalp. However those who have some hair can wear these easily.

INSIDE WEFTING: An cost effective alternative to a hand-tied ventilation. This machine-sewn fiber weft allows for softer napes and the ability for hair to lay flat in the back and nape.

BLEACHED KNOTS -The latest innovation in ventilation these days are called bleached knots. As the name is self-explanatory, these knots are put through a delicate bleaching process after being tied to the base with extremely tiny half knots. This removes most of the dark color and leaves a virtually invisible knot that really appears to be growing right from your scalp!

BLENDING -To achieve the most realistic color graduations in a final wig, hairpiece, or extension, factories will mix or 'blend' multi-colors of fiber together.

TOUPEE CLIP: These clips have been around a long time. They are sometimes referred to as "snap clips" or "snap lock clips," and are often called 6 finger clips because they actually have 6 little metal "fingers" that hold the hair when snapped shut. For added security, this small clip with grooves is sewn into the base of a wig cap, add-on, fall, or partial. They come in several sizes and colors. One must be careful when removing the wig from their head and carefully remove the hair that may still be in the clip or they will rip the hair. They are a wonderful adhesive, if you are careful and patient.

FINGER FLEX CLIP: The latest innovation in clip attachments. These wig clips are attached to polyurethane backing that wig tape can be adhered to for further security, and easily moved to different areas on the cap. There is the consensus that the clip should be moved on a piece every 5-6 weeks to lessen the stress on the follicle attached to the clip.

QUICK TOUCH CLIPS: A daily attachment; an alternative to clips that uses Velcro technology to adhere to the hair and adhesive backing to adhere to any hair system. Perfect for those who don't want wear metal or plastic clips

BANANA COMB: A banana clip is a long, 2-part, plastic hair clip with teeth on the inner side of each part that grasp the hair and snap closed at the top. Many wig companies take these clips and attach hair to them in various lengths and styles. When a person's own hair is pinned or pulled back in a short ponytail and the banana clip hairpiece is snapped closed over it, it creates the illusion of a ponytail or bustle effect down the back of the head.

BUTTERFLY CLIP: Pressure sensitive butterfly shaped comb with interlocking teeth that attaches under your own hair. Simply press to open the teeth of the clip and it's ready to be inserted into your own hair.

ROOT CRIMPED: The hair is crimped at the base of the cap to create more "lift"; height and volume in the piece.

VELVET COMFORT BAND: To enhance comfort and security, 1" to 1½" of soft velvet-like fabric is placed at the inside front of wig cap.

VELCRO° SIZING ADJUSTMENTS: Two Velcro° tabs placed at the nape allow you to adjust your wig for a more comfortable fit.

STRETCH RIBBON LACE: Used in the lining of a wig cap to add stretch and security.

FLEXIBLE, OPEN EAR TABS: A soft piece of metal that allows to adjust the piece closer to the scalp for a more secure fit and to contour the face at your temple.

CUTICLE: The cuticle is the outer layer of the hair follicle. It has three layers: a cuticle (the outer layer), a cortex (the middle layer containing keratin, moisture and melanin, which gives it its color), and a medulla, which is the center of the hair shaft.

TYPES OF HAIR COMBS:

RAT-TAIL: A standard rat-tail comb measures from 8 to 10 inches in length. It is known for being accurate in sectioning the hair, hence, the comb was designed with very fine and closely apart teeth while the pointed end's like that of a straightened rat's tail, intended for pulling sections of hair. This tool is also essential for putting hair extensions and performing chemical treatments.

WIDE-TOOTH: Wide-tooth comb is used for detangling hair after a bath or shower with teeth designed well apart. It helps avoid hair breakage and serves all types and textures of hair. Perfect for preventing frizz in synthetic hair.

TEASING: Big hair or teased hair originated during the 50's era. This iconic hairstyle was made famous by tons of hairsprays and the ever dependable, teasing comb! Its teeth are close to each other, perfect for creating volumes in the hair. The ends of this comb can be used to pick up streaks of hair precisely.

REGULAR COMB: The regular comb has teeth that are not so wide nor near to each other. It is somewhat in the middle between the wide-tooth and the rat-tail. This is used to detangle locks before and after shower. This kind of comb is ideal for straight and wavy hair.

PICK: Pick Comb is great for styling: especially lifting the hair away from the head. Similar to the teasing comb, pick combs can also help in adding volume to hair.

Sex, Wigs and Whispers

ATTACHMENT SYSTEMS AND PRODUCTS FOR WIGS: Tape, adhesives or other ways to attach hair temporarily or semi-permanently.

ADHESIVE: Available in either liquid roll-on or tape form, aids in securing wig to scalp.

HAIR ENHANCER: Often referred to as "Top Piece", Topper, "Topette®" or Halo. Designed to work with your own hair to add volume.

HAIR EXTENSIONS: Hair strands, either one piece or multiple strands that are designed to add length and volume to your own hair that are either sewn in or made with clips to attach to existing hair. May either be temporary or semi-permanent and are available in synthetic or human hair.

HEAT RESISTANT HAIR: This is a special blend of fiber that is heat resistant and will allow you to use heat appliances such as a blow dryer or hot rollers. Keep in mind that hair that is not attached to the head has no natural oils, nor does it breathe. Less heat is suggested to extend the shelf life of the piece. We suggest you use Caruso Steam Curlers more often than electric heated accessories. When applying heat on human hair, for added protection I suggest using a Thermal Protectant spray.

HAIR FRAMES: Your classic headband with heat resistant hair attached that can be designed to work with the front of your hairline.

GLASS LOOPS: A flexible opening in the cap to allow for a more comfortable and secure fit when wearing eyeglasses. Few manufacturers can do this correctly as everyone's facial structure and measurement is individual, there is no one measurement that works completely.

PINKING SHEARS: Scissors whose blades are a zigzag pattern instead of a straight edge; especially designed for cloth or any fabric to prevent from easily fraying. Perfect to use when cutting lace front pieces to give a more natural appearance.

BONDING: A process by which a hair piece is glued on to the head for a period of time.

EXTENDED WEAR: Are bonded pieces that are meant to stay on for 2-6 weeks at a time without before needing to be taken off and cleaned, giving the scalp a moment to breathe before being replaced and re-glued.

STAYS: A small piece of metal placed at the temple and nape to secure the fit of the wig.

VELCRO CLOSURES: Located at the nape of most of our wigs, these closures adjust easily to help create a custom fit.

WIG LINER: A lightweight mesh or nylon cap worn underneath the wig to help keep hair in place.

OPEN EAR TABS: Flexible material at the ears which allow you to adjust and contour the wig to your face around the temple area.

PRE-STYLED WIG: The wig has been pre-cut, shaped by the manufacturer.

READY-TO-WEAR WIG: Refers to a wig or hairpiece that is pre-styled. What you see is what you get.

NAPE: The area at the back of the neck at the base of the skull where the bottom of the wig fits against the head.

Sex, Wigs and Whispers

HIGHLIGHTS: The process of using lighter contrasting colors of hair to create a sunlit appearance. They may be light or heavy streaks blended throughout the entire wig or just at the front. and sides Highlights are generally used less than a 50-50 proportion.

LOWLIGHTS: The process of using darker contrasting colors of hair to create dimension. They may be light or heavy streaks blended throughout the entire wig or just at the front, and sides Lowlights are generally used less than a 50-50 proportion.

PROFESSIONAL STYLING: Most wigs will require some cutting and styling to create the individual wearer's desired effect. A professional wig stylist who can help you achieve your look and teach you how to use various approved wig care products is preferred. Remember, you would be best to take off too little than too much as it will not grow back.

ALOPECIA: A medical term meaning hair loss. Alopecia [alo-pe-shah] loss of hair; baldness. It is determined that millions of people around the world are afflicted with alopecia. The cause of simple baldness is not yet fully understood.

ALOPECIA AREATA: Alopecia Areata: A patchy type of hair loss in sharply defined areas, usually the scalp or beard due to an autoimmune condition; a common cause of hair loss. It often starts with one or more small round bald patches on the scalp and can progress to total body hair loss (alopecia universalis). Alopecia areata affects approximately two percent of the global population overall, including more than 30 million + women in the United States alone. This common skin disease is highly unpredictable and cyclical. Hair can grow back in or fall out again at any time and the disease course is different for each person.

Glossary

ALOPECIA TOTALIS: An uncommon condition characterized by the loss of all hair on the scalp. The cause is unknown and the baldness is usually permanent. No treatment is known.

ALOPECIA UNIVERSALIS: Alopecia Universalis is a medical condition involving rapid loss of all body hair, including eyebrows and eyelashes. It is the most severe form of alopecia areata.

ANDROGENETIC ALOPECIA: A condition where hair is lost due to a genetic predisposition.

Androgenetic Alopecia (alopecia androgene´tica) is a progressive, diffuse, symmetric loss of scalp hair in both men and women. In men, this condition is also known as male-pattern baldness. In men it begins in the twenties or early thirties with hair loss from the crown and the frontal and temple regions, ultimately leaving only a sparse peripheral rim of scalp hair. In females it begins later, with less severe hair loss in the front area of the scalp. In affected areas, the follicles produce finer and lighter terminal hairs until terminal hair production ceases, with lengthening of the anagen phase and shortening of the telogen phase of hair growth. The cause is unknown but is believed to be a combination of genetic factors and increased response of hair follicles to androgens.

Hair is lost in a well-defined pattern, beginning above both temples. Over time, the hairline recedes to form a characteristic "M" shape. Hair also thins at the crown (near the top of the head), often progressing to partial or complete baldness. The pattern of hair loss in women differs from male-pattern baldness. In women, the hair becomes thinner all over the head, and the hairline does not recede. Androgenetic alopecia in women rarely leads to total baldness. In women, androgenetic alopecia is associated with an increased risk of polycystic ovary

Sex, Wigs and Whispers

syndrome (PCOS). PCOS is characterized by a hormonal imbalance that can lead to irregular menstruation, acne, excess body hair (hirsutism), and weight gain.

ANAGEN EFFLUVIUM: Pathologic loss of anagen or growth-phase hairs. Classically, it is caused by radiation therapy to the head and systemic chemotherapy, especially with alkylating agents.

CICATRICIAL ALOPECIA (alopecia cicatrisa´ta): Irreversible loss of hair associated with scarring, usually on the scalp.

CONGENITAL ALOPECIA (alopecia congenita´lis): Congenital absence of the scalp hair, which may occur alone or be part of a more widespread disorder.

ALOPECIA LIMINARIS: Hair loss at the hairline along the front and back edges of the scalp.

MOTH-EATEN ALOPECIA: Syphilitic alopecia involves the scalp and beard that occurs in small, irregular scattered patches, resulting in a moth-eaten appearance.

SYMPTOMATIC ALOPECIA (alopecia symptoma´tica): Loss of hair due to systemic or psychogenic causes, such as general ill health, infections of the scalp or skin, nervousness, or a specific disease such as typhoid fever, or to stress. The hair may fall out in patches or there may be diffuse loss of hair instead of complete baldness in one area.

TRACTION ALOPECIA: Traction alopecia is the loss of hair caused by physically stressing and putting tension on the hair. Certain hairstyling including hair weaving and corn rows that were done too tightly can cause this type of hair loss.

AUTOIMMUNE CONDITION: Arises from an overactive immune response of the body against substances and tissues normally present in the body. In other words, the body actually attacks its own cells.

COMFY GRIP: This is a product designed to wear under wigs to keep them from shifting.

HYPERTHYROID CONDITION: An overactive thyroid condition.

HYPOTHYROID CONDITION: An under-active thyroid condition.

NON-SLIP MATERIAL: A special material that is built into the wigs to keep it from sliding and shifting

NON-SURGICAL HAIR REPLACEMENT PRODUCTS: Any type of wig, hair piece, or cranial prosthesis, etc.

TRANSPARENT TAPE: This is a tape that is used to adhere to the poly-skin like material and scalp to provide extra security so that the wig will not shift. A small percentage of people are allergic. However, to be sure you will not have an adverse effect to the tape, take a small piece and place it on the top of your hand or arm for five (5) minutes. Make sure your skin is dry with no oils or moisturizer or the tape will not adhere correctly. If he area starts to itch, swell or burn, or when you remove the tape it is bright red, you are most likely allergic to the tape and should seek the advice of an experienced dermatologist for suggestions on another type of tape or adhesive.

POLYURETHANE TABS: An incredibly resilient, flexible, and durable manufactured material that is used on the perimeter of a cap to adhere tape or glue to for stronger security.

HEAT SENSITIVE MATERIAL: This is a material that is used in the construction of a wig cap to prevent the cap of slipping and shifting. The material adheres to the head due to the heat that is released from the scalp producing a suction-like effect.

LACE TAPE: Lace tape can be used for daily wear and is placed in small amounts to secure the lace material to the cap. It is suggested to use a citrus removing solution to remove the residual adhesive from the tape as it protect the lace material from ripping or shredding.

SYNTHETIC ROOT COLORS: The synthetic fiber is darker at the root area and is lighter toward the ends.

THIN SKIN MATERIAL: This is a material that is used in a specially designed cranial prosthesis. It has a very natural appearance and is extremely fine and thin. It produces an effect as if hair is naturally growing from the scalp. This is often used for bonding a wig onto the scalp with a specialized bonding glue that will hold it in place for six weeks before it will need to be taken off, cleaned and reattached with fresh glue.

LETTER OF MEDICAL NECESSITY: This is a letter that is sometimes required by insurance companies in order to reimburse patients for a "medical cranial hair prosthesis." Patients can request a letter of necessity from their physicians to provide to the insurance company.

MEDICAL CRANIAL HAIR PROSTHESIS: This is a specially designed wig with special features for comfort, natural appearance, and special needs of the medical hair loss patient.

WIG INSURANCE REIMBURSEMENT INSTRUCTIONS: Your physician will provide you with a prescription for your wig known in medical terms as a *Full Cranial Hair Prosthesis*. Be sure to call your insurance provider and find out if your policy includes this coverage (including the specific reimbursement amount and number of wigs). (See Appendix A: "Insurance Reimbursement")

Glossary

Remember Girls, We're More Than Just Hair!

CPSIA information can be obtained at www.ICGtesting.com
Printed in the USA
BVOW07s2052140116

432559BV00033B/244/P

9 780986 284243